PRAISE FOR

Black Fathering and Mental Health

"Dr. Michael Hannon and his colleagues have broken new ground with a unique and timely contribution to the literature of Black fathering and anti-racism. Through their lived experience as sons and fathers, combined with their education and experience as mental health counselors, they are transparent, vulnerable, proud, reflective, articulate, committed, engaged Black men who thoroughly disrupt the racist trope of the absent Black father. Their lived experiences are diverse and reflective of the broad spectrum of family constellations in our society. I read this manuscript as an Arab American, having raised two Biracial Black children with special needs. The fears expressed about their children experiencing the dangers of racism and white supremacy resonated deeply in my heart from when I held my children for the first time. Each contributor includes reflections on how counseling helped or could have helped their fathering. Hannon's concluding chapter is actionable recommendations for counselors and other mental health professionals for working with Black fathers. In sum, this book will instruct and inspire the reader with the resilience and determination of Black men and fathers."

—Robert Naseef, PhD, Alternative Choices, Psychologist, Author of *Autism in the Family: Caring and Coping Together* and *Special Children, Challenged Parents: The Struggles and Rewards of Raising a Child with a Disability*

"*Black Fathering and Mental Health* is a rich, nuanced account of the reality of Black fathering in the context of their families, neighborhoods, villages, and larger society. While reading, you feel like you are sitting next to these men as they share their innermost thoughts and feelings, and their lessons learned, about the strengths, challenges, and triumphs of Black fatherhood. As a counseling psychologist, I see this book as an inspiring look inwards into one's own community, telling the story as only insiders can. It is an essential text for counselors and any mental health professional working to understand and support Black fathers or fathers-to-be. In fact, I would argue that it is a must read for anyone who has Black men and boys in their lives."

—Muninder Kaur Ahluwalia, PhD, Professor, Montclair State University, Author of *Taking Action: Creating Social Change through Strength, Solidarity, Strategy, and Sustainability*

"Rarely have the voices of African Americans fathers been recognized. This text highlights the lived experiences of courageous African American men. Each chapter provides a window into the inner lives of African American fathers in ways that help professional counselors directly meet their mental health needs. This needs to be a required text for practicum and internship counseling courses."

—Carla Adkison-Johnson, PhD, LPC, Department Chair and Professor, Western Michigan University and Editor-in-Chief, *Journal of Multicultural Counseling and Development*

"This beautiful book makes me want to be somebody's father. It overflows with love, impressive vulnerability, inspiring examples, and useful guidance. It is a must-read for every Black man who is or aspires to be a father, as well as everyone who aims to effectively support them."

—Shaun Harper, PhD, Clifford and Betty Allen Professor, University of Southern California, Author of *College Men & Masculinities: Theories, Research and Implications for Practice* and *Advancing Black Male Student Success from Preschool Through PhD*

Black Fathering and Mental Health

This book is part of the Peter Lang Education list.
Every volume is peer reviewed and meets
the highest quality standards for content and production.

PETER LANG
New York • Bern • Berlin
Brussels • Vienna • Oxford • Warsaw

Black Fathering and Mental Health

Black Fathers' Narratives on Raising Their Children Across the Family Life Cycle

Edited by
Michael D. Hannon

PETER LANG
New York • Bern • Berlin
Brussels • Vienna • Oxford • Warsaw

Library of Congress Cataloging-in-Publication Data

Names: Hannon, Michael D., editor.
Title: Black fathering and mental health: Black fathers' narratives on raising their children across the family life cycle / edited by Michael D. Hannon.
Description: New York: Peter Lang, 2022.
Includes bibliographical references.
Identifiers: LCCN 2021044295 (print) | LCCN 2021044296 (ebook)
ISBN 978-1-4331-9309-5 (paperback)
ISBN 978-1-4331-6080-6 (ebook pdf) | ISBN 978-1-4331-6081-3 (epub)
Subjects: LCSH: African American fathers—Mental health services. | African American men—Mental health services. | African American families—Psychological aspects. | Parenting—Psychological aspects.
Classification: LCC RC451.5.B53 B53 2022 (print) | LCC RC451.5.B53 (ebook) | DDC 362.2089/96073—dc23
LC record available at https://lccn.loc.gov/2021044295
LC ebook record available at https://lccn.loc.gov/2021044296
DOI 10.3726/b19422

Bibliographic information published by **Die Deutsche Nationalbibliothek**. **Die Deutsche Nationalbibliothek** lists this publication in the "Deutsche Nationalbibliografie"; detailed bibliographic data are available on the Internet at http://dnb.d-nb.de/.

80 Broad Street, 5th floor, New York, NY 10004
www.peterlang.com

This book is dedicated to the people who have required, nurtured, and inspired my Black manhood and my Black fatherhood across our family life cycle. They are Dr. LaChan V. Hannon, Nile Joyce Marcelle Hannon, and Avery Mekhi Hannon. I love you with all I am, and any measure of success I have experienced in life as a partner and father is because of you. Thank you for the people you have been, the people you are, and the people you continue to become. I am grateful for all of it and pray we have long years ahead to enjoy and love each other.

This book is dedicated to my fathers, mothers, and family. To my biological parents—Rev. Byron and Annette Hannon—I am so proud to be connected to you. Thank you for your love without condition or pretense. To my parents in love—Coach Neil and Dr. Beverly Hutton—I've told you that I never saw true forgiveness in action until I met you. Thank you for accepting me and allowing me into your lives. And to my sisters—Stephanie, Lia, and Kori—I am ever grateful for my relationship with each of you individually and collectively.

Finally, this book is dedicated to the Black men who have and continue to father their children with commitment, fidelity, and intensity. I appreciate you, as does our community. We are not the same without you, and I hope you find your own narrative in the pages of this volume.

Table of Contents

List of Illustrations

Foreword

REV. BYRON L. HANNON

When Michael called me because there was an issue on which he wanted my opinion, I did not expect him to ask me to write this foreword. I assumed that he, my son, was interested in my thoughts on something that mattered to him. It would not have been the first time we have had this kind of conversation; it is a natural extension of our relationship, one that I still cherish even though he is well into his adulthood.

I have written thousands of pages as a student, a leader in a corporate setting, a minister, and a blog writer. I have helped an author-friend, serving as an unofficial editor of her book. I was not expecting this; being asked was nowhere on my mental radar, but I am honored to offer some thoughts with the hope that it will be a worthy opening to the stories that follows.

All of you readers should understand that I cannot help but to be biased in my comments; Michael Hannon is my son. I ask you to be forbearing, believing that you will eventually make your own judgment about this entire work and by, extension, him. I have known my son from that early October morning in his hospital delivery room. Since that day, he and I have spent countless hours together during every stage of his life whether in the context of family interactions, church fellowship, academic life, and during the times when he and I were each other's sole company. I fondly recall those many hours in the car headed to and from wrestling matches and baseball and soccer games, working in the yard around the house, and more recently having breakfasts at a local diner. I have viewed each of these times, particularly when he was a boy, as opportunities to listen and, where I felt it was needed, to impart some bit of knowledge (and hopefully, wisdom) because I knew the day would come when he would need to stand on his own in a world that would seek to sway him toward its various and often conflicting directions, a world which would not always value him as a person.

I have watched my son develop his ability to understand, express and pursue his passions. I have watched as he developed the ability to weather storms. I have watched him become his own man. I have watched him mature and grow older as I have grown old. One thing I can say through all of this is he has always had my deepest respect. And my love. I like the man Michael has become and is becoming. I say the latter because I believe health requires continual growth that is independent of age.

As with all people and relationships, there have been bumps in the road, some significant enough to wrestle with openly and others more suited to silent waiting. I recall the concern I had when he announced his decision to transition from a career focus in student life to the academic side of the academy. My wife, Michael's mother, has long been fond of saying, "Sometimes you have to take a step backward in order to take two forward." Was he ready to take the backward step, to make the sacrifices, the big sacrifices, to attain his goal? Had he counted the cost? It turns out, much to my relief and gladness, he was ready; he had not only counted the cost, he paid it. Of course, none of this was done in a vacuum; he had and has a supportive wife, children, extended family, and friends as encouragers and helping hands. They are individually and collectively worthy of acknowledgement. I am deeply grateful for them and all who helped him on this journey. Now, I have the privilege of watching my son, a father, a Black father, pour his life into his children, my grandchildren.

This book is about Black fathering and, therefore, is first and foremost about fathering in all of its forms. There comes a time in every parent's life when it is necessary to stand back and allow your child to follow their dreams and for others to invest in your child's life as well as have the opportunity to make assessments about the person in whom you have invested so much. Those evaluations about competency, commitment, passion, preparedness, and core integrity occur implicitly and explicitly, over and over again in an unceasing rhythm. It certainly has been my privilege and my responsibility to play a significant role, along with others, in preparing my children for this. This earnest attempt is what I believe what fathers should do. It is a return- producing investment, not an expense, and this book is one visible manifestation.

Compassion is a word that comes to my mind often. I think of this, not as solely a *feeling*, but as a heartfelt *response* to becoming cognizant of a legitimate need that cannot be met without some intervention. To borrow and slightly amend a common phrase, I believe compassion begins at home. Who more than our children are in need of continual intervention to meet needs that cannot be met independent of parental engagement? As I write this, I am thinking of a little three-year-old boy I was asked to lay hands on and bless yesterday at the conclusion of a church service in Philadelphia. He was there with his grandmother and aunt, two women of Afro-Caribbean descent. Who besides them are going to be there to guide him through the developmental and maturing stages of his life? Who is going to be there to teach him how to be comfortable in his own skin and to understand that his desires cannot be met at the expense of others? Who is going to teach him to respect women, whether they be his sisters, his mother and grandmothers, his aunts, his cousins, his teachers, his classmates, and the adult women who will show up later in his life? Who is going to teach him how to handle success and disappointment and even failure? Who is going to tell him when he is wrong? Who is going be his cover for the arrows which inevitably will be shot at him? Who is going to be his champion and chief encourager? Which man (or men) will play these important roles in his life? An engaged dad, an uncle, a teacher, a coach, a clergyman, perhaps all of the above; he needs their compassion so that he can stand and grow into an emotionally healthy Black man.

While an undergraduate student in the early 1970s, my dorm roommate, an education major, was questioned by a White professor in a sociology course, "Mr. S___________, what do you consider yourself to be, Black or Afro-American?" My roommate immediately replied, "I consider myself B_______," speaking his first name. It may not have initially occurred to this professor that my friend was, first and foremost, an individual with agency. Thankfully my roommate, at age 19, was self-aware and secure enough to reframe the issue to fit *his* terms, not those of someone who did not know him. In the thinking of this prof, my friend's individuality was less significant than his group membership. Aside from the teaching agenda of this probably well-meaning professor, a prevailing motive for many, I believe, is to align with the socially dysfunctional orientation that categorizes people into groups and then designates them as allies or enemies, as superior or inferior by comparison. Why? Because it is easy to do and is consistent with the paradigms of racism along with other forms of oppression. A major challenge of being Black in this nation is an outgrowth of this dysfunction in which inferiority is assumed, causing the need for books like this to be written.

I am a preacher and pastor by calling and vocation. And because my ministry passion is spiritual formation, formation as a general concept holds much appeal for me. We all are the beneficiaries of the formative inputs from our parents and other sources be they positive and healthy or less so. These inputs add definition to our identities and not only shape us, but they also play a role in what we reproduce in those who follow us. We can take our lesson from nature: fruit produces like fruit. Health promotes health. The opposite is prone to be true as well. Our formation almost invariably translates to our children and forms a cornerstone in their lives. We know there are no perfect people and necessarily, there are no perfect parents, no perfect fathers. We need them and we need others. Each of us needs to experience the blessings that come to us from others who give us something of themselves. I have been incredibly blessed by my father and by other men and women older and wiser than me. I have gained and grown because of their investment in me. The times when what they shared was difficult for me to receive have often turned out to be exactly what I needed and grew to appreciate the most.

What might have happened to me if, after suffering a disastrous 7th grade year and facing the anger and frustration of my own father for bringing Cs and Ds home for the first time, had Mr. Prater not intervened? One of the few Black male teachers in my middle school, Mr. Prater informed me on the first day of 8th grade that he was going to "intellectually emancipate" me. As a 13-year-old, that was cryptic to me although I did sense care and concern. Mr. Prater pushed me *and* encouraged me all school year and I recovered. My grades improved and I regained my confidence in time in to enter high school. He knew what I needed. Mr. Prater, though long deceased, remains one of my heroes.

The musical artist Taj Mahal penned a song entitled *Clara (St. Kitts Woman)* on one of his early albums (Mahal, 1974), a paean to his grandmother. One lyric phrase referring to his grandmother is striking:

She would hold you, love you and scold you,
Making sure she told you
They will never know what it is you need

The truth, the unfortunate truth, is that Black children have needs that non-Black adult authority figures have little to no awareness and are ill-equipped to meet because of the structural racism of our world that does not touch and infiltrate their lives as it does Black men, women and children. They cannot relate and this lessens their ability to lead. Beyond this is the issue of widescale disinterest which has to be acknowledged. I know enough about the educational process to know that we learn what we want to learn. Is it absolute truth that "they" will they never know; that "they" cannot know? I cannot say this is as an axiom, but I know from experience, observation and the valid testimony of others that so many are not seeking to know. This is the epitome of privilege; when members of a dominant (i.e., more influential) group can choose when and how they engage with those who are less dominant and influential because of structural forces. Fully engaged Black fathers (and mothers) whether they be in the home or elsewhere (custodial or non-custodial as used by some of the book's writers) like Mr. Prater, are the ones who know what is needed and can and are needed to play a fundamental role in the development of children.

You may remember the scene from *Roots* (both the book and TV series) when Omoro Kinte held his infant son, Kunta, up to the starry night sky and said, "Behold, the only thing greater than yourself!" a ritual Kunta years later repeated with his baby daughter, Kizzy (Haley, 1976). In the latter example, this physically enslaved but mentally free Black father took this first step to imbue his daughter with a sense of her incalculable worth just as his father had done for him. I am not a professional educator; I am a pastor who believes in the inherent worth of every human being because they are bearers of the *Imago Dei* (Image of God). For this reason alone, every child, including every Black child, deserves to have the best opportunity discover their gifts, their talents and passions, their purpose without the need to bear the additional burden of systemic racism imposed upon them. Given our world, perhaps that is too optimistic a goal which speaks to the need for texts like this.

I love my children. They are unique and special to my wife and to me. There is nothing unique about this testimony, however; it is a near universal attitude and that is a great thing. That said, regard for our children, our Black children is not universal. They need champions; they need protectors; they need those of us who have walked the path, seen and experienced its pitfalls and who can guide them safely. They need fathers and mothers and others who will bless them with compassion from the day they are born until the day there is nothing left to give them. My prayer is that this book is a source of light and clarity in a world often filled with shadows and darkness and is a help to those who participate in this ministry of guiding.

Rev. Byron L. Hannon, father of Stephanie, Michael and Lia and the son of Lafayette, who was the son of Claude, who was the son of John, who was the son of Green, who was the son of Lucinda, a slave.

Acknowledgments

I am deeply indebted to many people for this project coming to fruition. To the team at Peter Lang Publishing, led by Patty Mulrane and Dani Green, thank you for your support through this process. I look forward to the possibility of working together moving forward. I need to acknowledge my Montclair State University Department of Counseling community. Thank you to all of the students, faculty, and staff who challenge and support me to be the best version of myself in my role as a faculty member, adviser, and supervisor. I appreciate all of you. I want to especially thank Natalie Nieves and Raymond Blanchard who unselfishly worked with and for me as doctoral fellows during the evolution of this project. Thank you.

I want to acknowledge my clinical supervisor, boss, and sister-friend, Dr. Ebony White, with and for whom I have the pleasure of working. 'Preciate you, doc! To Dr. Robert Naseef, I am especially grateful for your friendship and mentorship. Thank you for being you. I am grateful for our ongoing work with and for fathers of individuals with autism. I can't express all of the gratitude and love I have for my #homeplace team. You know who you are and I'm not the same Black man without your friendship. Thank you. Finally, I am happy and grateful to acknowledge the Black fathers, aspiring Black fathers, and generous community members who contributed to this volume. Thank you for partnering with me to offer an unheard, undervalued, misunderstood AND absolutely needed narrative about us and those like us. Ase'.

List of Abbreviations

NCC	National Certified Counselor
LAC	Licensed Associate Counselor
LPC	Licensed Professional Counselor
LMHC	Licensed Mental Health Counselor
ACS	Approved Clinical Supervisor
PhD	Doctor of Philosophy
EdD	Doctor of Education

Introduction

MICHAEL D. HANNON, PHD, LAC, NCC

This creation of this edited volume has a few inspirations. First, it is inspired by my family, which includes my biological and chosen kin. All of them are sources of inspiration for me and provide a level of support, critical feedback, encouragement, and motivation that is immeasurable. Second, it is inspired by Black fathers. Many of us are keenly aware of how Black men, and particularly Black fathers, are dangerously and consistently presented in various media as absent, disengaged, and dangerous. It is an absolute privilege—with the help of my dear friends and colleagues—to offer this counter-narrative. Families and Black fathers' roles therein change constantly. However, changing family constellations and roles does not equate to absence or disengagement. The Black men—fathers and aspiring fathers—featured in this volume are as diverse as the roles they assume in their families and communities. Third, it is inspired by the counseling profession. The American Counseling Association (ACA) is the "world's largest association exclusively representing professional counselors in various practice settings" (ACA, n.d.) and defines counseling as "a professional relationship that empowers diverse individuals, families, and groups to accomplish mental health, wellness, education, and career goals" (ACA, n.d.). Although professional counseling is allied with, and informed by, other mental health professions (e.g., psychology, social work, psychiatry), it is unique based on four beliefs about counseling practice and the people served by counselors (Neukrug, 2016). First, professional counselors practice from a wellness perspective. We prioritize identifying and leveraging what is well in those seeking counseling services over focusing on impediments to wellness. Second, professional counselors use a developmental perspective in their work with individuals, groups, and families. That is, we believe that many of the challenges besetting those seeking services are developmental in nature. There are some normative experiences individuals and communities share that include, but are not limited to raising children and adolescents, educational experiences, entering and leaving committed relationships, and aging. Counselors understand there are challenges—and sometimes crises—during these important developmental milestones, which inform how we help.

Third, professional counselors value prevention and early intervention. While all challenges are not preventable, we are deeply concerned and moved to take preventative action or develop early interventions to mediate problems we know can possibly be debilitating for individuals, families, and communities. Fourth, and finally, professional counselors believe and support client empowerment (Neukrug, 2016). We believe that individuals seeking services generally have the capacity to live successfully without being dependent on counseling services. Consequently, we work to help clients identify and leverage their strengths, assets, and capital to be productive and lead lives that they see as fulfilling.

ORGANIZATION AND CONTENT

What follows in the chapters of this book are accounts of Black fathers and aspiring fathers sharing—in narrative form—how we have fathered our families at different points across the family life cycle (Carter & McGoldrick, 1989). It is informed by the important scholarship of John McAdoo (1993), who argued that understanding Black fatherhood must be considered in light of the systems that influence how Black men father. He shared that a comprehensive understanding of Black fatherhood recognizes the influence and effects of racism on Black fathers' ability to fulfill their assumed or assigned roles (McAdoo, 1993). It's my contention, and those who have contributed to this volume, that fatherhood influences men's mental health. Researchers have documented this influence in positive ways like facilitating more healthy behavior in men (Garfield et al., 2010) and in stressful ways such as having to renegotiate roles when each new child arrives, leading to both extreme satisfaction and potential distress (Shezifi, 2004), which Chin, Daiches and Hall (2011) described as "finding a place" in the new family system. We also know and appreciate that fathers' presence and engagement uniquely influence their children's development, including their socio-emotional development (Easterbrooks & Goldberg, 1984); cognitive development (Shannon et al., 2002), and linguistic development (Conner et al., 1997). We offer first-person reflections of the triumphs, elation, fear, and disappointments associated with being Black fathers to our children in what we know is an anti-Black world.

My colleagues and I have provided in-depth accounts of our experiences to accomplish three separate but related goals: (1) raise our voices to share our challenges and victories fathering our families; (2) illuminate the circumstances that may (or should) have dictated the need for counseling support and how it was (or could have been) helpful; and (3) provide counselors and allied mental health professionals recommendations for effectively working with Black fathers and their families. What makes this book important is because there has not been a volume that has intentionally asked and answered these questions of Black fathers. It is also unique because the Black fathers who have contributed to this book are all professional counselors and counselor educators who offer a dimension of personal, critical reflection, and insight that is paramount for counselors and other mental health professionals.

All chapter authors discuss their fathering experiences at different points across the family life cycle. As you have hopefully already read, my father, Rev. Byron Hannon offers his reflections in the foreword to this text, reminding us all about the how critical Black fathers and other fathers are in the emotional and spiritual formation of their children. Then, in the first two chapters, Dr. Tyce Nadrich and Dr. Alfonso Ferguson write separately about expectant fatherhood. The perspective in the first chapter is offered by Dr. Nadrich's experiences as a straight, cisgender Black man. The second chapter is presented by Dr. Ferguson from his perspective as an Afro-Caribbean, same-gender loving, Black man who aspires to father children with his husband. The following chapter is provided by Dr. Kent Butler, who provides readers his own insights and experiences on fathering his Black daughter to support her mental wellness and school readiness.

Dr. Sam Steen follows in chapter four with his reflections on Black fathering as an engaged, non-residential parent. Dr. Linwood Vereen offers insight about the joys and challenges of fathering biracial children. In chapter six, Dr. Eric Williams presents his narrative about being the Black father of two autistic children, followed by Rev. Robert Rogers' deeply reflective chapter on fathering his adolescent children. I present my lessons learned on trying to support my adolescent children's mental health needs, and Mr. Rodney West walks readers through his experiences fathering his adolescent son—and relatives—in preparation for post-secondary success. Dr. Gelawdiyos Haile, Dr. Amber Haley, Dr. Amber Norman, and Dr. Butler offer insights about being the adult children of Black fathers. I offer a summative account of recommendations and considerations for counselors and allied mental health professionals treating Black fathers in the next chapter. And, Dr. Ivory Toldson closes the text with a poignant afterword.

In each chapter, the authors respond to four overarching questions. They are: (1) who/what were biggest influence on your fathering?; (2) what did/does

Black fathering look like for this time in your life, in light of your child's/children's needs?; (3) what kind of counseling support do/did you need (or get) to navigate this time in your life and what did you learn as a result?; and (4) what should counselors know about counseling Black fathers during this time frame? What follows are honest and compelling narratives that we believe are equal assets to our professional and home communities.

Michael D. Hannon, Ph.D.
July 2021

REFERENCES

Carter, E. A & McGoldrick M. (1989). *The changing family life cycle: A framework for family therapy.* Gardner Press: United States of America

Chin, R., Daiches, A., & Hall, P. (2011). A qualitative exploration of first-time fathers' experiences of becoming a father. *Community Practitioner, 84*(7), 19–23.

Conner, D. B., Knight, D. K., & Cross, D. R. (1997). Mothers and fathers scaffolding of their 2-year-olds during problem-solving and literacy interactions. *British Journal of Developmental Psychology, 15*(3), 323–338. doi:10.1111/j.2044-835X.1997.tb00524.x

Easterbrooks, M. A., & Goldberg, W. A. (1984). Toddler development in the family: Impact of father involvement and parenting characteristics. *Child Development, 55*(3), 740–752.

Garfield, C. F., Isacco, A., & Bartlo, W. D. (2010). Men's health and fatherhood in the urban Midwestern United States. *International Journal of Men's Health, 9*(3), 161–174. DOI: 10.3149/jmh.0903.161

Neukrug, E. S. (2016). *The world of the counselor: An introdcutoin to the counseling profession* (5th ed.). Cengage: Boston, A.

Shannon, J. D., Tamis-LeMonda, C. S., London, K., & Cabrera, N. (2002). Beyond rough and tumble: Low-income fathers interactions and children's cognitive development at 24 months. *Parenting: Science and Practice, 2*(2), 77–104.

Shezifi, O. (2004). When men become fathers: A qualitative investigation of the psychodynamic aspects of the transition to fatherhood. *Alliant International University, San Diego. ProQuest Dissertations and Theses,* Retrieved from http://search.proquest.com/docview/305047797?accountid=13158

CHAPTER ONE

Expectant Straight Black Fatherhood

TYCE NADRICH, PHD, LMHC, NCC, ACS

FATHER PROFILE

Tyce Nadrich has been partnered with Josie since 2005 and married since 2012. They were expecting the birth of their first child in June of 2020. Tyce is a Licensed Mental Health Counselor in New York state, Board Certified Counselor, and Approved Clinical Supervisor. He received his PhD in Counseling, is a full-time professor of Clinical Mental Health Counseling, and operates a private practice working predominantly with People of Color, specifically adolescents and young/middle-aged adults.

I AM A MAN RAISED BY WOMEN

More specifically, I am a man who was raised by Black women. These women are the foundation of everything I know about being a parent and father. I grew up in South Jamaica, Queens with my mother and older brother. Our community was firmly in the lower-middle class; we all lived in houses, but a lot of us received some form of assistance or aid like reduced lunch, WIC, or something similar. Most of us were Black and Brown; either shortly before my family moved in or during my "too young to remember" years (likely a little of both), most of the White residents moved out of this section of South Jamaica, an exodus that can be described as White Flight (Kye, 2018). The near-nonexistent presence of fathers was another commonality within the neighborhood I spent my first 18 years.

The first friend I remember having, a Latina girl about nine months older than me who lived directly across the street, had just one of the two fathered households. Sadly, the only prominent memory I have of him is his death during my late childhood or early adolescents. The other fathered household was far more distant. We lived in the middle of a block that had 42 houses on it—we were number 19, to be exact—and this home was on the corner. For a child, this was a world away, far out of ear-shot of my mother calling me home during the times before cell phones. What I remember about him was that he was the quintessential "man's man." He was tall, bald, had a deep voice, and had tools (he may have been a plumber, by trade), and he had a tone that when he said something, it was not to be challenged. This family divorced and moved during my adolescent years.

The families I was closest with were led by women—Black and Brown mothers with children and intermittently present or absent fathers and father-figures. They formed a community of sorts among each other, one that I cannot imagine was formally created or had discussed and defined rules. If the mother from two doors down, who had two children of her own, a son approximately my brother's age and a daughter roughly mine, caught me doing something I should not have been, she punished me herself. Then, she would send me home with instructions to tell my mother what she caught me doing. This, of course, resulted in another punishment. These women were unflinching, omnipresent, and unwavering; they were also loving, nurturing, and supportive. As I reflect on what influenced my impending role as a father, this is the foundation, most saliently my mother.

My mother always told me "if you're not White, you're Black." She instilled in me that race influenced how the world sees you. I interpreted this as a lesson to ensure I did everything in my power to not allow my Blackness to hold me back. She always wanted me to "speak properly." This did not apply when I was with my neighborhood friends or close family, but whenever we were in less familiar environments, she never allowed me to use slang. In hindsight, those less familiar environments were usually predominantly White environments. Anytime she heard me curse she would make me get the dictionary and find three to five new words—depending on her mood, I assume—to replace the curse in that specific sentence. I think my mother wanted me to know how to code switch, or to be able to shift my language and overall presentation so I would be more likely to navigate predominantly White environments (Cross & Strauss, 1998). My mother also masked any financial troubles we had throughout my childhood. As a child, eating lasagna and other pasta-based dishes most nights a week felt fancy, even luxurious. Also, my mother stocked up on all different kinds of pasta when the boxes were on sale for a dollar plus whatever coupon she had. In fact, while I was working as a counselor in juvenile detention, a young boy shared with me that he was looking forward to going to "Welfare Camp." "What is Welfare Camp?," I asked him. He looked at me like I was stupid, lifted his shirt, and exposed his White undershirt with a very familiar and somewhat-nostalgic logo. That evening, I called my mother and asked her, "Did I go to Welfare Camp?" My brother and I were none-the-wiser.

My mother taught me to be Black. She protected me from the world and myself. She hid things from me that would only cause pain and highlighted things that maximized my exploration and enjoyment of the world. She loved me and made sure I knew that she loved me. She pushed me to be better than her. This is the type of father I want to be.

Men and my development

I have no memory of my mother and father married or cohabitating. My early memories of my father involve mostly pleasantries: playing and watching baseball, going to Blockbuster Video and watching movies at his Brooklyn apartment. However, I only saw my father on weekends. I want to say it started with weekly visits and slowly became less frequent, but I am not entirely sure. What I can say is that as a young child, when I was with my father I felt attended to, cared about, and appreciated. However, by late childhood my father started dating someone which culminated in their moving to Northern Connecticut. I believe my father tried his hardest to balance his new responsibilities with fatherhood. He was a part of a blended family now and lived 120+ miles away; there was, undoubtedly, less time (and possibly resources) to engage with me and my brother. Plus, as my brother and I grew older, our desire to spend time with our parents waned as it does with many adolescents, resulting in even less opportunity.

There are two other fatherhood lessons I can attribute to my father: speaking up and expressing emotions. My father is White, and I have always felt like an outsider within my father's family. My Blackness was never more apparent to me throughout my childhood than it was at a Thanksgiving dinner table with at least 12 other White relatives. My brother and I were the only splash of color in the room, and it was evident both visibly and culturally. As I got older, I was able to recognize clear disparities in how (my brother and) I were treated with my father's family. Most of the interactions were small and subtle, and would clearly be described as racial microaggressions in today's vernacular (Sue et al., 2007).

To my knowledge, my father never publicly or privately confronted his family on their interactions with me. I am confident I would have benefitted from this if it happened, or had he even spoken to me directly about it. Maybe things could have changed if there was an increased dialogue about these interactions. Maybe my relationship with this side of my family would be different today had we addressed things more explicitly. Maybe I would have felt validated that these occurrences were real and not my own fabrications, relieving some of the pressure I felt to try to understand them. At minimum, I think I would have felt comfortable sharing how I felt at these events with my father had he overtly broached the topic. Consequently, remaining reticent about social tensions affecting my daughter is not acceptable in my fathering approach. I need her to know that I see her navigating the world and that I want (and intend) to be along for that ride.

My father was—and still is—an emotionally expressive man. He did not ascribe to very traditional ideas about masculinity. He was not the stoic, silent type; he shared his feelings and showed his vulnerabilities. As a self-described emotional individual, my father's modeling made me feel more comfortable with my feelings and expressing them, something I intend to do for my daughter as well. I want to model for her that feeling and expressing emotions is both normal and healthy. Further, I want her to see that I feel too, both with her and for her.

Most of the other lessons I learned from the men in my life were a result of negative experiences, unfortunately. The lessons were positive, but the experiences were not. I often encountered men who would tell me what I should do, yet I watched them do the exact opposite. "Don't do drugs" while they would smoke marijuana; "treat women with respect" while using derogatory terms about women or being overt abusers. Lesson learned: model what you want your children to understand; don't fall into the hypocrisy of "do as I say, not as I do." I remember hearing the men in my life question why I didn't come to them sooner, or why I didn't share with them what I was going through. I felt burdened bringing my problems to the men in my life, as if I were imposing my issues onto them when they didn't ask for it. Lesson learned: intentionally and actively be present with your children; don't wait for them to seek you out for their needs. I had (and continue to have) diverse interests. I wanted to play baseball and basketball, but I also wanted to do gymnastics, be a part of the band, be a peer mentor, and play video games. I felt that the men present throughout my childhood often emphasized my athletic endeavors and minimized (or even ridiculed) my other interests. I assume that there are interests that I had as a child that I was so ashamed of or embarrassed about that I never shared them and have likely forgotten about them entirely. Lesson learned: allow your children to express themselves organically; don't force your perceived missed opportunities or individual priorities onto them. My mother always spoke to me for who I was: an ambitious, emotional, smart, and impulsive biracial Black boy. I do not think the men in my life ever saw me as holistically as my mother. They may have seen parts (such as my Blackness or my maleness) but never the full picture. I never felt like a man was "my guy," my role model, or the person I looked up to or aspired to be. Lessons learned: teach your children what it means to exist in a world with their unique identities (e.g., what it means to be Black); don't let them believe the world is blind to race or sex and everyone will treat them fairly or equally. Show them that Black men can be caring, loving, present, supportive, and everything they need; don't let them absorb the egregious narratives about Black men. There will likely be enough narratives of insufficient fathers or father-figures my daughter will encounter, so I intend to be the embodiment of the counternarrative.

WHAT DOES BLACK FATHERING LOOK LIKE FOR THIS TIME IN YOUR LIFE?

It took us eight months to get pregnant. I expected (we both expected) it to happen immediately. I remember we decided we were going to start trying right before we went on a vacation to the Caribbean in May of 2018. We had a whole plan:

1. As soon as we return from vacation, we remove Josie's birth control.
2. No immediate expectations; it may take 2–3 months for Josie's body to adjust to the change (although I'm sure we were both secretly hoping it would happen immediately).
3. Get pregnant in August or September.
4. Bank Josie's vacation/holiday time and we'll both be home for the entire summer.

Our naiveté was very real. A friend once told me "God doesn't care about your plans." We were pregnant in January, and we had a miscarriage in late February.

We decided to go to a fertility specialist in July, one year after we started trying. A month's worth of tests concluded we were both carriers of Spinal Muscular Atrophy, "the second most common fatal autosomal recessive disorder after cystic fibrosis, affecting approximately 1 in 6000 to 10,000 live births" (Muralidharan et al., 2011, p. 3). In short, there's a 25% chance our child would have this condition, 50% chance they would be an asymptomatic carrier, and 25% chance she would be condition-free. We were told the only way to guarantee not passing the disorder to our children was through in-vitro fertilization; the doctor also provided us a quote of a little over $20,000 for the procedure, with no guarantees of success, of course.

And the way our bank account is set up …

About one week later, while exploring more affordable solutions, my wife spontaneously and unexpectedly told us we were pregnant. Twelve weeks later we were told our daughter is an asymptomatic carrier; the amount of relief that accompanied that phone call was incomprehensible. Prior to that call I was going through the world with weighted clothing, half-inserted ear plugs, and foggy glasses. In an instant there was catharsis, relief, and clarity, and I began to assess what would have been (the previous 12 weeks) and what was coming.

Fathering at this time in my life can only be described as before and after learning my child was healthy. Before that phone call, fatherhood was about survival. I was perpetually distracted, indefinitely worried, and—if I'm being honest—probably clinically depressed. I did my best to support my wife; I put her needs above everything else, including my own. I neglected my physical and mental health, and probably was not as supportive as I wanted to be for my wife—I was operating at a significantly lower capacity than I normally could. Fatherhood at this time was a perpetual struggle of trying to accept that I was powerless to do anything to remedy the situation.

"GOD DOESN'T CARE ABOUT YOUR PLANS"

Fathering after learning my daughter was healthy changed significantly. Of course, supporting Josie was my ongoing duty and privilege. We had a new list now, but everything focused on preparation—birthing plan, birthing class, infant care class, baby shower planning, building a nursery, baby-proofing the house, finding a pediatrician, planning for leave, exploring childcare options, adjustments to finances, etc. I'm confident many of these thoughts arise for most, if not all, parents. However, some I think are unique to me, being Black, and my historical and current socioeconomic status. How can I teach my daughter to navigate the predominantly White neighborhood we live in? The predominantly White schools she will likely attend? Can I protect her from racism? Sexism? How do I teach my daughter the lessons I learned through my experiences? I grew up in Queens, attended schools in disinvested communities, got into fights, etc. I don't want her to experience these things directly, but I want her to have the information I possess from my trials and tribulations.

Fathering is also learning as much as I can from the fathers I know. I'm fortunate to have a good number of Black fathers in my life as an adult, people I view as mentors and big brothers. Every chance I get, I speak with them about what it means to raise Black babies. I ask my friends and family about their childrearing experiences; I'm doing my best to learn from those that are already doing it. I'm also taking classes every chance.

WHAT KIND OF COUNSELING SUPPORT DO/DID YOU NEED (OR GET) TO NAVIGATE THIS TIME IN YOUR LIFE AND WHAT DID YOU LEARN AS A RESULT?

I did not seek or obtain professional counseling services. However, I absolutely should have. I struggled with self-blame and feeling powerless a few months into trying to conceive. I assumed something was wrong with me. I did not differentiate our conception struggles from my self-worth. My feelings of inadequacy were compounded when we learned about carrying Spinal Muscular Atrophy. Feelings of powerlessness were exacerbated.

Not only was I incapable of conceiving a child, but even if I could, there was no guarantee of health.

I experienced the most difficulties throughout the three-month period while we were pregnant but did not know if our baby was healthy. The limbo state was unbearable at times. I was irritable, sad, had difficulty sleeping and focusing on tasks, and had difficulty enjoying life.

In hindsight, I probably met the criteria for clinical depression

I think I avoided counseling for two reasons. I felt selfish going to counseling and I felt compelled to keep my struggles private. My feelings of selfishness were grounded in the fallacy that any energy or attention taken away from my pregnant wife was a waste. I convinced myself that her needs were exceptionally important; therefore, my needs were diminished. And to be clear, this was in opposition to what Josie wanted.

She urged me to seek support and help, I just didn't listen.

I wanted all the focus to be on her; I thought to myself, "If I feel this way and I'm not even carrying the baby, imagine how she feels." The unfortunate consequence was that in my efforts to focus entirely on her, I neglected myself and was insufficiently resourced to best support her, which only fostered more guilt and negative emotions.

I am naturally more inclined toward privacy over sharing; I'm more introverted than extroverted, and prefer small, close-knit groups than larger ones. Congruently, I held our intentions to get pregnant and all subsequent events closely. Instead of counseling, I leaned on very few friends throughout the process. Although I shared with these friends what was happening, I don't think I even truly spoke in depth about my struggles. And although I did this intentionally, I think I was partly hiding from my own feelings of embarrassment or shame. I am the second to last of my childhood friends to have children and part of me wondered if my waiting affected my ability to conceive. Similarly, in my wife's culture (she is of Dominican heritage), we were expected to have children many years ago, especially considering how long we have been together. In fact, some (if not all) of her family assumed we were never going to have children. A part of me worried that we had made a mistake in waiting as long as we did, even though I am exactly the same age as my mother was when I was born.

Throughout this process, I think I learned two overarching lessons: I have less control than I want and it's OK (and probably for the best) to ask for help and support. Learning that I have very limited control is probably a salient lesson for any parent to learn. I had little to no control over when our child would be conceived, whether she would be healthy, and when she decides to bless us with her arrival. Similarly, I will not have much control over how the world interacts with my daughter and my influence toward the person she will become are unknown. I gather that part of becoming a father is learning to focus on the things I can control, make efforts to influence the areas where I have varying degrees of control, and minimize my energy toward things that are entirely out of my control. Relatedly, learning to ask for support will be essential as a father. I didn't seek support throughout the early stages of our pregnancy, and I wasn't the best version of myself. I do not want to make the same mistakes, ongoing. Also, I want to model for my family that asking for help is an appropriate and necessary action to take.

WHAT SHOULD COUNSELORS KNOW ABOUT COUNSELING BLACK FATHERS DURING THIS TIME FRAME?

Foremost, internalized bias and racism is real and can affect Black fathers. Counselors should be aware of the pressures that may be on Black men to be present, attentive fathers. There are many negative stereotypes attached to Black fathers; the racist and biased narratives of the "dead-beat dad" and the Black father who doesn't take care of his children are prominent (Cooper et al., 2019). While I am confident in my ability to be an effective father, I also feel heavy pressure to do so. I am terrified to give anyone space to pass judgment on my fathering. This is partly, if not primarily, motivated by not wanting to be labeled as a subpar Black father. My standards are already quite high and the additional pressure to combat stereotypes can be exhausting at times. Counselors should be aware of the pressure expectant Black fathers may feel to combat the narratives of broader society.

Somewhere at the back of my mind, I internalized inaccurate messages about conception and fertility. I remember feeling like the world lied to me when we were having difficulties conceiving. I felt like I was taught that the moment you have unprotected sex, someone will get pregnant. I am confident many men experiencing difficulties with fertility question themselves. However, I think counselors should be aware of the unique role race can play in Black men approaching fatherhood, insofar as the pressure to be an attentive and present father in conjunction with the issues any potential father may face.

Lastly, I think counselors should be aware of the importance of community for expectant Black fathers. The phrase "it takes a village" resonates among parents, including Black fathers. Community can be pivotal in successful and healthy parenting, and counselors should be mindful to foster Black fathers to seek community support as needed. I recall attending an infant care class recently, and I wondered why we were the only People of Color in attendance. The class was free, offered on a Saturday, and in a location accessible by public transit or driving. Yet, in that moment I felt lonely, and the feeling did not assuage until I spoke with my extended village of Black fathers. This experience may be a microcosm of what Black fathers experience at their children's schools or extracurricular activities, depending on their community. Counselors should be mindful to encourage Black fathers to find their community and use the support they afford.

EPILOGUE: COVID-19

I initially finished writing this chapter in January of 2020. I began doing final revisions in April, deep in the heart of the COVID-19 pandemic. Although this section was not part of my initial draft, I felt my experiences here were too salient to not include.

On the evening of March 22, 2020, New York State enacted a plan limiting the frequency of social interactions in an effort to slow the spread of COVID-19. Things were changing in the weeks before this announcement; my college moved to online instruction in early March and my private practice moved to telehealth services shortly thereafter. As COVID-19 began infecting New York State, I only thought of this through my role as a counselor, professor, and citizen. I was concerned for the welfare of my clients and the transition to telehealth services. I was worried for my students that may lose their jobs and/or internship placements. I was anxious for all my friends that were essential workers and my wife, a pregnant ICU nurse, in a hospital that was slowly filling with COVID-19 patients. However, my role as a father became apparent when our obstetrician's office informed us that I was not permitted to attend appointments anymore. I took great pride in being there for every doctor's appointment, every sonogram, every baby-related event. And now I'm not allowed to attend any of them, ongoing, indefinitely. Shortly thereafter, we began to hear that hospitals were restricting people from accompanying laboring mothers, and we confirmed that the hospital we intended on delivering with restricted all persons from labor and delivery. I was existing in a society that was focused on what was deemed essential. Essential workers must continue to work and essential businesses remain open. People were discouraged from leaving their homes except to attend to their essential needs. Within this, the message was loud and clear to me: fathers are not essential to the birthing process of their children.

New developments and adjustments occurred throughout the weeks thereafter. I drive my wife to the doctor's appointments and wait in the car. Sometimes we would video chat during the appointment so I'm there in some capacity. Other times, I'm content just being nearby in the parking lot. Since my wife is perfectly capable of driving herself to these appointments, I'm not sure whether my presence is more supportive of myself or of her. I like to think it's the latter or, at minimum, it is in support of both of us. Yet, I feel guilt when I think my waiting in the parking lot is for my sole benefit. Although I have made improvements toward attending to myself during this time, I have more work to do. In the final days of March, the governor of New York ordered that hospitals permit at least one partner for laboring mothers, so I will be in the room when my daughter is born. However, we have had to change hospitals because the place we intended on going to forces all partners to leave once the mother and baby are moved to the postpartum unit (even if the partner tested negative for COVID-19 and never left the mother's side). We've had to cancel our baby shower and all child-related courses have been moved online. However, writing this chapter and putting a voice to my experiences has brought me great catharsis and increased confidence to share my needs with others. Although fatherhood continues to be a perpetual struggle of trying to accept that I am powerless in many situations, as I move toward acceptance, I am less burdened by the things I cannot control and better resourced to focus on the things I can.

REFERENCES

Cooper, S. M., Ross, L., Dues, A., Golden, A. R., & Burnett, M. (2019). Intergenerational factors, fatherhood beliefs, and African American fathers' involvement: Building the case for a mediated pathway. *Journal of Family Issues*, *40*(15), 2047–2075. https://doi.org/10.1177%2F0192513X19849629

Cross, W. E., Jr., & Strauss, L. (1998). The everyday functions of African American identity. In J. K. Swim & C. Stangor (Eds), *Prejudice: The Target's Perspective* (pp. 267–279). Academic Press.

Kye, S. H. (2018). The persistence of white flight in middle-class suburbia. *Social Science Research*, *72*, 38–52. https://doi.org/10.1016/j.ssresearch.2018.02.005

Muralidharan, K., Wilson, R. B., Ogino, S., Nagan, N., Curtis, C., & Schrijver, I. (2011). Population carrier screening for spinal muscular atrophy: A position statement of the association for molecular pathology. *The Journal of Molecular Diagnostics*, *13*(1), 3–6. https://doi.org/10.1016/j.jmoldx.2010.11.012

Sue, D. W., Capodilupo, C. M., Torino, G. C., Bucceri, J. M., Holder, A. M. B., Nadal, K. L., & Esquilin, M. (2007). Racial microaggressions in everyday life: Implications for clinical practice. *American Psychologist*, *62*(4), 271–286.

CHAPTER TWO

Aspiring Black Fatherhood from a Same Gender Loving Lens

ALFONSO FERGUSON, PHD., LMHC, NCC

FATHER PROFILE

I am a licensed mental health counselor in the state of New York, and, among other things, I am a Black, same gender loving (SGL), Afro-Caribbean, cisgender man navigating the rocky terrain that is the United States (US). In my work as a clinician, I have been privileged to work with predominantly Black and Brown individuals living in New York City and surrounding communities. Moreover, I specialize in working with queer people of color (QPOC). As a clinician and member of the QPOC community, I have noticed and recognized that QPOC generally experience a series of challenges, trauma, and resiliency within their family systems. For many of the Black men I have worked with, they were taught about fatherhood, manhood, and masculinity from their fathers, father figures, and older male family members in their lives. As an adult Black SGL man, I am often unlearning and relearning what it means to be in relationship with other men, whether straight or SGL. In addition, I am often working with Black SGL male clients to reconcile the teaching they learned as children about fatherhood, manhood, and masculinity. Through a Black queer lens, I intend to identify the ways my intersectional experiences have prepared me for the father I hope to become in the near future.

INFLUENCES OF FATHERING

Researcher Diana Baumrid's seminal research study from the 1960s identified multiple parenting styles, including authoritarian, authoritative, and permissive (Baumrid, 1967, 1971, 1991). Authoritarian parents can be described as parents who are very strict, controlling, and inflexible (Baumrid, 1967). Authoritative parents may be parents who retain authority and control but are also warm and communicative (Lamb & Baumrind, 1978). Authoritative parents are often seen as demanding but also responsive. Permissive parents, on the other hand, may present with low demands or control but are also present and responsive to the needs of their children (Baumrid, 1967, 1971, 1991). Researchers later added a fourth parenting style, permissive-indifferent or uninvolved, which is described as absent, neglectful, and inattentive to the needs of their children (Maccoby & Martin, 1983). In thinking about the different parenting styles, I am immediately inspired to identify parenting or fathering style I aspire to be and why. My father was and is an authoritative parent, and our values are consistently in alignment.

Although my expectant fathering has been influenced by many experiences, my initial reaction is to name my father as the biggest influence on my fathering style. My father, Alfonso Ferguson, Sr., wears many hats in our familial system. He is an uncle, cousin, brother, stepfather, grandfather, and father.

From him, I have learned that fathering is serious business, but you do not have to take yourself too seriously.

There are many things my father taught me growing up, and if I am honest, he still teaches me things on a regular basis. There are several core tenets of fathering I have learned directly and indirectly from father. Those core tenets of fathering include communication, trust, and unconditional positive regard.

Communication is my father's superpower and one skill I aspire to master when I become a father. My father has developed this unconventional skill of constantly communicating and remaining present in the lives of all his family members. I have not quite figured out how he does it, but he speaks to and checks in with all of his nine children as well as the four mothers of his children, all while being gainfully employed. Might I add, his children and their mothers are spread out across three states and two countries. I often joke with friends, "If I don't speak with my father for more than 48 hours, he would file a missing person police report." Today, I am still convinced he would do this. Through his tenacity to stay connected and communicate with everyone in his life, I learned the value of talking to family and building and maintaining relationships.

Trust is key in any relationship. My relationship with my father helped me to define and identify trust. Through authentic experiences with him, I have been able to cultivate trust with others. As a child, I experienced trust through security.

My father made sure my basic needs were met regularly, but he also deemed himself trustworthy as he was integrous with all his commitments. Another core tenet of my father's fathering style was unconditional positive regard. If my father had a career in the counseling profession, he would absolutely subscribe to the Rogerian counseling aesthetic (Rogers, 1979). Though my father set boundaries and had high expectations for his children, he also showered us with unconditional support and attention. Some research has shown that Black fathers who have a pattern of showing intimate affection or unconditional positive regard can contribute to higher self-esteem, emotional well-being, and improved mental health in their children (Fagan, 2000; Hossain et al.,1998; Lewis-McAdoo, 1979). Black fathers showing intimacy and affection can be described as soft masculinity, which is an East Asian ideology of an alternative construction of masculinity compared to the Western patriarchal approach (Ainslie, 2017; Ayuningtyas, 2017; Jung, 2011). As a result of my father's approach of soft masculinity from an Afro-Caribbean man, our relationship and my emotional well-being is forever strengthened.

In addition to my biological father, there are other men in my life who have been instrumental in shaping my fathering characteristics today. One such person is my high school track and field coach, Horace Ruddock. Coach Ruddock was my coach from the age of 13 to 18. In my life and the lives of hundreds of student athletes, Coach Rudduck was an otherfather. Otherfathers can be described as men or authority figures who provide holistic care, support, parenting, modeling, and life coaching to others (Brooms, 2017). Based on Baumrid's parenting style, Coach Ruddock would be an authoritarian father. As a coach and otherfather, he had high hopes, expectations, and demands for us. For almost six years we trained and competed 11 months a year (i.e., indoor season, outdoor season, summer season, cross country). My biggest takeaway from Coach Ruddock was his selflessness and familial sacrifice. Coach Ruddock treated our small group of athletes as if we were his own children. He made sure we ate before and after every practice no matter our familial financial circumstance, and he transported us to and from practice and track meets (i.e., local, regional, out of state). Coach Ruddock was never paid by any of our families for his services as a coach and otherfather. For me, Coach Ruddock is the epitome of selfless fathering. I aspire to be as selfless in my fathering as Coach Ruddock was in his otherfathering practices.

Lastly, my most recent influence on my fathering style would be my interactions with Gregory "Nana" Russel. Nana, as we call him, is an older Black (i.e., mid-60s) SGL man that I met in my late 20s. Gregory earned the name Nana as a reflection of the Black queer ballroom scene where individuals were often forced to create chosen families that mimic traditional family structures (i.e., mother, father, sister, and brother). I remember we were at the dining table eating dinner Gregory cooked. As we joked about our age difference, we decided that he was too senior to be my house mother so instead it would be more fitting for him to be my house grandmother, also known as Nana. He embraced the new name with laughter and excitement. From then on he began to introduce us as his children. Our shared community embraced the name Nana, but it was also a testament to the many people in his life in which he had been otherfathering. It is always interesting when he introduced me to his friends that have known him for most of his life. He would say, "Hi ____, This is my son Alfonso!" Like a proud parent, he would then report my gifts, talents, and accomplishments. Nana subscribes to a more permissive parenting style (Baumrid, 1967), which is possibly influenced by my age and independence. I would describe Nana as a true nurturer. Nana's love language is acts of service, and this rang true every time we shared the same space (Chapman, 1992). Nana enjoyed cooking and being of service in any way he could. Moreover, Nana nurtured my journey of reconciling my intersectionality as a Black SGL Afro-Caribbean man.

Nana identifies as gay, and he lives his life unapologetically, loud and proud. His way of being was and is contagious.

As Black men, we often draw from our direct and indirect experiences of how to navigate our Blackness, manhood, masculinity, and paternity. The aforementioned men provided me with salient ingredients with which to cultivate my fathering style. Those ingredients include communication, trust, unconditional positive regard, selflessness, and nurturing. In the words of the African philosophy Ubuntu, "I am, because we are. Since we are, therefore I am" (Mbiti, 1969, pp. 108–109).

BLACK FATHERING AT THIS TIME IN MY LIFE

As I contemplate fatherhood and begin to position myself to engage in the process of seeking surrogate support or adoption, I also then reflect on how this experience may affect my identity as a Black SGL man. I imagine there will be many emotions that arise. Even in the act of envisioning what that journey can look like and how it may feel when I arrive at my fathering pinnacle, I am filled with a mix of emotions, such as excitement, anxiety, sadness, and fear.

I am excited because I have always imagined myself as a father,—so much that for many of my younger siblings I am a father figure or paternal representation in their lives. For instance, there is a 23-year age gap between myself and my youngest sibling. Due to the limited presence of his biological father, I have assumed some paternal responsibilities, such as attending parent/teacher conferences, creating reward systems, assuming some disciplinary responsibilities, instilling life lessons, and providing love and support. I am excited and fulfilled by the young man he is becoming. At the tender age of eight, it is clear that he will grow up to be a curious, expressive, sensitive, caring, and honest man. As a parental figure in his life, I cannot help but to think about what he will need during his adolescent years and how I can contribute to his growth and progression as a contributing citizen of the world.

In addition to being excited about the potential of being a father to my own child and a father figure to my younger siblings, there is also some anxiety about officially taking on the responsibility of being a father.

I am anxious because of the societal pressures that are imposed upon Black fathers.

Society has stigmatized Black fathers as being absentee parents or parents with minimal engagement (Richarson, 2019). I worry about becoming a statistic as a father—whether its overcommitting to career pursuits and not allowing time for familial bonds or underutilizing the patience required to form authentic connections with an infant. Moreover, there is some concern about being a Black SGL father and the challenges and/or microaggressions that may arise. For instance, if we choose to conceive a child through surrogacy, who will be the biological father? If myself or my husband are not the father, will it be my child or our child? In the medical field, options for surrogacy, and in-vitro fertilization advance, male SGL parents are becoming more able to incorporate both fathers' genes into the unborn child. For instance, hip-hop fitness sensation Shaun T and his husband, who happens to be white, conceived twin boys through surrogacy. It is evident that one child is of mixed race while the other is white. Though this alleviates some anxiety about being the biological father and having a blood bond with my child, there are provoking thoughts. Those thoughts include, what kind of world will my child live in? As a Black child will they experience racial equity or liberation? As a father, will I be present, loving, caring, and attentive? As a counselor, I recognize that these anxious thoughts are normal for any parent expecting, particularly parents of color. It is important to allow myself the opportunity to experience and challenge these thoughts and trust that I will always make the best decision within my power for myself and my child.

Furthermore, there is some sadness and fear about bringing a Black child into this world. Given the current state of the world (i.e., Coronavirus Disease 2019 [COVID19], resistance to racism), it is abundantly clear how disproportionately marginalized Black people have been and continue to be. The Black community in the US is negatively affected by COVID-19 at disproportionate rates. According to the Center for Disease Control and Prevention (CDC), at the peak of the first wave of the global pandemic 92.3 Black persons per 100,000 died of COVID-19 compared to 45.2 white persons (CDC, 2020). The CDC (2020) highlighted living conditions, work circumstances, underlying health conditions, and lower access to care as a few of the leading causes for inordinate racial disparities of

COVID-19 deaths. COVID-19 is essentially a microcosm of the racial inequity happening on a national and global level.

To father a Black child would mean bringing a child into a world where their race places them at an immediate disadvantage. To father a Black child would mean one of my first responsibilities is to teach them how to survive as a Black person. That survival is dependent on helping to prepare them for ongoing and difficult conversations about how others may treat them because of their race. It means always having some level of healthy paranoia because you can never feel too secure about your positionality at work or in life because it can be taken away from you at any given moment. My ideals of fathering during this time are slightly tarnished because to bring a Black child into this world during this time may mean that their life and my legacy is subject to annihilation because of the color of their skin.

COUNSELING SUPPORT

My father always says, "sometimes coffee, sometimes tea!" For me, that translates to some days are good and you are equipped with all the necessary tools needed to take on the world, but there will be times when you are not prepared and you manage your experiences the best you can. As a Black SGL aspiring father, there are several support systems I have sought out and put in place. In recent years, I have positioned myself to be around more Black SGL couples in committed relationships (i.e., marriage) with similar aspirations of one day becoming parents. We have created a support system for one another. As Black SGL aspiring fathers, we intentionally discuss strategic planning on the best approach to becoming fathers in the near future. In addition, we have discussed potential challenges of becoming Black SGL dads in the current sociopolitical climate. Though not the traditional form of counseling support, this support group of Black gay aspiring fathers has helped tremendously on this road to fatherhood.

Having a support system of Black gay men with similar familial goals has helped my partner and I to strategically conceptualize fatherhood. As a group, we have discussed the different options for pursuing fatherhood, such as adoption, foster care, surrogacy services, and traditional methods of child conception. Research has shown that gay and lesbian couples experience greater discrimination and more challenges when adopting or fostering children (Weiner & Zinner, 2015).

Though there is no empirical research to suggest that same-sex parenting is less successful, there seems to be a healthy societal resistance to LGBTQ parents (Biblarz & Stacey, 2010; Bos, van Balen, & van den Boom, 2007; Weiner & Zinner, 2015).

Moreover, I imagine there are additional challenges for the intersectionality of being both Black and same-sex parents.

In doing our research, we have learned that surrogacy is another potential option. In recent years, it has become more apparent that many gay, and some straight, couples are choosing to obtain a surrogate to carry their child. Gay celebrities, such as Shaun T and his husband as well as Bravo's millionaire listing franchise celebrity Fredrik Eklund and his husband, conceived through surrogacy. As an aspiring Black SGL father, I admire the ways Shaun T and his husband are raising their children. It is important to note that surrogacy can be expensive and risky. My husband and I have researched surrogacy options and cost in the US. After a brief Google search and reviewing a few surrogate support websites, we quickly learned that the financial commitment would be upwards of one hundred thousand dollars or more. Amongst our group, we have also discussed seeking international surrogate support. Friends of friends of ours utilized a surrogate organization based in Africa. Though the couple experienced some turmoil during the process, they now have twin girls who are healthy and thriving.

In addition, many gay couples also consider utilizing the traditional form of child conception. My partner and I have been approached once or twice by our lesbian friends about the possibility of conceiving a child together. Moreover, we have made agreements with straight women in our lives to one day conceive a child together. For us, it was not the right time and, in some cases, not the right set up or prospective mothers' circumstances change and childbearing is no longer an option. This is a challenge most gay and lesbian couples face when trying to conceive a child in a traditional framework. It has to be the "perfect storm," meaning the persons involved have a shared vision of the process, procedure, journey, and life of the child(ren). In many cases, we have discussed questions like—how will you be involved? Are you a donor or do you want to be an active parent in the child's life? In the support group, we have also explored the feelings (i.e., sadness, frustration, anger, hopelessness) that may come up when an attempt to conceive in a traditional framework does not come to fruition.

In my counseling practice I have worked with numerous SGL individuals and couples who navigate the pre-parenthood phase of parenting. In working with a lesbian couple, I learned that they have had similar challenges with choosing a donor or paternal contributor. The couple expressed wanting to conceive through utilizing the turkey baster method. According to Thompston (2017), the turkey baster method can increase a woman's chance of conceiving by 22% and is significantly more cost effective than in-vitro fertilization. For this and other SGL couples, the challenge has been having the initial conversation, curating a mutually beneficial parenting environment, and identifying an appropriate donor profile. Failing to conceive can impact all persons and relationships involved.

COUNSELORS SUPPORTING SGL ASPIRING BLACK FATHERS

Due to the intersectionality of Black SGL fathers, there are several things that counselors may need to recognize and understand about their Black SGL aspiring fathers' lived experiences. Black SGL men have multiple marginalized identities and have historically experienced challenges in the various communities to which they belong. For instance, some Black men may be subject to racism in the larger systemic experience, heterosexism in the Black community, and objectification within the gay community. It is important that counselors are prepared to address the various ways Black SGL men experience oppression in addition to parenting challenges. In order for counselors to effectively support Black SGL fathers, it is vital they adhere to and honor the counseling profession ethical standards of the Multicultural and Social Justice Counseling Competencies (MSJCC; Ratts et al., 2015). The four developmental domains that are central to MSJCC are counselor self-awareness, client worldview, counseling relationship, and counseling and advocacy interventions (Ratts et al., 2015). As counselors, it is important to be clear about their positionality within these four domains as these are important to effectively support all clients, but especially clients who are multiply-marginalized such as Black SGL fathers. Subscribing to the MSJCC will support counselors in addressing their attitudes and beliefs, knowledge, skills, and actions.

As counselors, we can support Black SGL fathers on several levels: (1) individual, (2) family, (3) friends, (4) peers, (5) community systems, and (6) historical levels. On an individual level, counselors can encourage intrapersonal learning for clients to connect and understand how their different identities contribute to their challenges and resiliency as parents. Given the opportunity to focus on family, friends, and peers, counselors may support their clients in reconciling their interpersonal experiences and how it contributes to their overarching emotional well-being. Moreover, recognizing the ways community systems (i.e., school, spiritual institutions, public health systems, legal and economic resources, etc.) affect clients can help them navigate systems more effectively. Supporting clients through the community systems level may involve connecting clientele to resources and advocating for changes that marginalize diverse populations (Hays & Erford, 2018). Lastly, it is important to understand how SGL men and Black men have been historically oppressed, as well as the ways they have been resilient. All in all, it is of the utmost importance that counselors address all aspects of their clients' identities, environmental make up, and the stigmas associated with each area.

Moreover, it is important to recognize that Black SGL fathers are both resilient and marginalized. Black SGL fathers are resilient in that there are many obstacles that are overcome to reach a status of fatherhood. Personally, I experience racism, heterosexism, toxic masculinity, patriarchy, white supremacy, and systemic oppression on a regular basis. These experiences have equipped me with the necessary tools needed to withstand any oppressive experience. It is important for counselors to recognize this resilience and to approach the counseling relationship from a strength-based framework rather than a focus on deficits. In addition, it is important for counselors to not only create safe spaces but also allow clients opportunities to explore things that are pertinent and important to them. With this freedom of exploration, it is crucial that counselors do their own work to address any biases, stereotypes, stigmas, and assumptions they have about marginalized groups. Emotional harm is a direct ramification of counselors not addressing their own biases and stereotypes. At the core of adhering to MSJCC, counselors must be empathic and compassionate to the populations with whom they work, including Black SGL fathers.

CONCLUSION

The great Chinese philosopher Lao Tzo once said, "A journey of thousand miles begins with one single step." I have taken a few steps in this journey to becoming a Black SGL father. I am excited for what this experience will bring. I anticipate there being highs and some lows. My experiences with my biological father and otherfathers have equipped me with the necessary love, empathy, patience, tenacity, and perseverance that is needed to be the father I aspire to be. Black fathers and otherfathers are a gift from a higher power, and I look forward to being a gift to my child.

REFERENCES

Ainslie, M. (2017). Korean soft masculinity vs. Malay hegemony: Malaysian masculinity and Hallyu fandom. *Korea Observer, 48,* 609–638.

Ayuningtyas, P. (2017). Indonesian fan girls' perception towards soft masculinity as represented by K-pop male idols. *Lingua Cultura, 11*(1), 53–57. http://dx.doi.org/10.21512/1c.v11i1.1514

Baumrind, D. (1967). Child care practices anteceding three patterns of preschool behaviour. *Genetic Psychology Monographs,* 75, 43–88. doi: 10.1037/h0024919.

Baumrind, D. (1971). Current patterns of parental authority. *Developmental Psychology,* 4, 1–103. doi: 10.1037/h0030372

Baumrind, D. (1991). The influence of parenting style on adolescent competence and substance abuse. *Journal of Early Adolescence.*11, 56–95. doi: 10.1177/0272431691111004.

Biblarz, T. J., & Stacey, J. (2010). How does the gender of parents matter? *Journal of Marriage and Family, 72,* 3–22.

Bos, H. M. W., Van Balen, F., & Van Den Boom, D. C. (2007). Child adjustment and parenting in planned lesbian-parent families. *American Journal of Orthopsychiatry, 77,* 38–48.

Brooms, D. R. (2017). Black otherfathering in the educational experiences of black males in a single-sex urban high school. *Teachers College Record, 119*(12), 1–46.

Center for Disease Control and Prevention. (2020). Coronavirus disease 2019 (COVID-19): Racial & ethnic minority groups. https://www.cdc.gov/coronavirus/2019-ncov/need-extra-precautions/racial-ethnic-minorities.html.

Chapman, G. (1992). *The five love languages: The secret to love that lasts.* Northfield Publishing: Chicago.

Fagan, J. (2000). Afriacan American and Puerto Rican American parenting styles, paternal involvement, and Head Start's children's social competence. *Merrill-Palmer Quarterly, 46*(4), 592–612.

Hays, D. G., & Erford, B. T. (2018). *Developing multicultural counseling competence: A systems approach* (3rd ed.). Pearson: New York.

Hossain, Z., Field, T., Pickens, J., Malphurs, J., & Del Valle, C. (1998). Fathers' caregiving in low-income African-American and Hispanic-American families. *Early Development and Parenting, 6*(2), https://doi.org/10.1002/(SICI)1099-0917(199706)6:2<73::AID-EDP145>3.0.CO;2-O.

Jung, S. (2011). *Korean masculinities and transcultural consumption.* Hong Kong: University of Hong Kong Press: Hong Kong.

Lamb, M. E., & Baumind D. (1978). Socialization and personality development ın the preschool years M. E. Lamb (Ed.), *Social And Personality Development*,(pp. 50–67) Halt, Rinehart and Winsten: USA

Maccoby, E. E., & Martin, J. A. (1983). Socialization in the context of the family: Parent-child inter- action. In P. Mussen (Ed.), *Handbook of child psychology*, 4 (pp. 1—101). Wiley: Hoboken, NJ.

McAdoo. J. L. (1979). Father-child interaction patterns and self-esteem in Black pre-school children. Young Children, 34(2), 46–53.

Mbiti, J. (1969). *African religion and philosophy.* East African Education Publisher: Nairobi.

Ratts, M. J., Singh, A. A., Nassar-McMillan, S., Butler, S. K., & McCullough, J. R. (2015). Multicultural and social justice counseling competencies. Retrieved from https://www.counsel- ing.org/knowledge-center/competencies.

Richardson, S. (2019). Breaking the myth about Black fatherhood on this father's day. Chicago Reporter. https://www.chicagoreporter.com/breaking-myths-about-black-fatherhood-this-fathers-day/.

Rogers, C. R. (1979). The foundations of the Person-Centered Approach. *Education, 100*, 96–107.

Thompson, A. (2017). 'Turkey basting' increases a woman's chance of a successful pregnancy by 22% – and may be better than costly IVF. https://www.dailymail.co.uk/health/article-4738862/Turkey-basting-increases-chance-pregnancy-22.html.

Weiner, B. A., & Zinner, L. (2015) Attitudes toward straight, gay male, and transsexual parenting. *Journal of Homosexuality, 62*(3), 327–339. https://doi.org/10.1080/00918369.2014.972800

CHAPTER THREE

Black Fathering for Early Education Readiness

S. KENT BUTLER, PHD, LPC, NCC

FATHER PROFILE

Dr. S. Kent Butler, Jr. is a full professor and the Interim Chief Equity, Inclusion and Diversity Officer at the University of Central Florida. He is National Association of Chief Diversity Officer in Higher Education Fellow and American Counseling Association Fellow and current President- of the association. Among his many professional endeavors and accomplishments, Kent recently launched a podcast dedicated to equity, inclusion, and diversity entitled "Matters of Diversity with Dr. B." He loves to travel and enjoys spending quality downtime with his family and listening to old school, jazz, and gospel music. Kent Butler waited until after he was settled into his career before he embarked upon love and knew his eventual wife, Ann, was his soul mate. They married in July of 2011 and the following June, they welcomed their daughter Summer Joy. She is Kent's pride and joy, reminding him daily of the sacrifices of fatherhood and the love bestowed upon him from his own parents.

INFLUENCES ON MY FATHERING

I probably could never put into words what my parents mean to me, especially now that they are not physically on this earth with me any longer. I actually long for their presence and their loving ways. I miss so many things about growing up in the Butler household, memories like our Friday night fish dinners and other family traditions that were realities for me and my two sisters. I remember mostly the good times but also cherish the bad. I can look back and laugh at the punishment we received when we were clearly in the wrong. Perhaps painful then, but those punishments are experiences I grew from. They sometimes felt mean-spirited at the time, but those punishments kept us respecting our parents and on track for successful futures.

My father was our disciplinarian, and my mother was our nurturer. Together they were the best parents for whom I could have ever hoped. They provided me with a well-grounded childhood; I felt safe enough to ask for anything but needed for nothing. I always knew I had their love and the things that mattered. I learned through watching them how to love God, be fiscally responsible, and fend for myself. Though Christian in their values, they still let my sisters and me try different things throughout my life. They trusted me to be my own person. They celebrated my successes and my failures. They proudly empowered and supported me through my education even when they sometimes had no clue what I was doing as a graduate student.

They skillfully balanced setting boundaries while giving me opportunities to let me do my thing.

I have fond memories of both of my parents. I have particular memories of spending time with my father. He was a construction laborer and he would often take me on jobs with him, especially his weekend moonlighting gig with a furniture store to, among other things, breakdown and haul away cardboard boxes to the dump. Oh how I hated it! I felt he was tormenting me on purpose, being awakened early on Saturday mornings to ride around with him in his truck. I am sure some child labor laws were violated! I thought he was being mean, not wanting me to hang out and have fun with my friends on those days. He would pay me at the end of the day, and I would still be frustrated with him. But now I know he was creating time for me and for us. He was helping build my work ethic to be a responsible man and father. I'm eternally thankful for those memories. It was our time.

Even as a teenager and young adult, my father's influence on my fathering was tangible. I know he wanted me to appreciate the opportunities a college education could provide. But there was a semester when I took off from school and guess who helped me get a job, at his day job? Yup, my dad. And let me tell you, NOTHING makes you appreciate your education like construction work. The company hired me, paid me well, made me operate a jackhammer. Man, I couldn't get back into school fast enough! I smile knowing he wasn't disappointed because he wanted more for me. I wouldn't be me—as a Black man, a

Black father, a Black counselor, a Black leader—without his love and influence. I want that for my children and am that for my children.

Early counseling insights

I grew up not knowing the benefits of counseling and having someone to talk to about life. As a younger person and man, seeking a counselor was never on my radar. The only persons I knew to be counselors were our school counselors, and in my younger mind, they were the people who provided signatures for my course selections in high school. There were times when I could have benefitted from talking to a counselor to help me understand my father better. That could have been my school counselor or a counselor who worked in the community. Hindsight being twenty-twenty, I would have talked more to my school counselors; I bottled a lot in.

I believe that a counselor would have helped me find out sooner what my father was actually doing in raising my siblings and me. He was learning the ropes as he was going along due to losing his own father at an early age.

Had I known that these were the ways he showed me he cared, versus thinking he was being mean for no reason, I would not have rebelled so much against how he lived his life. I can admit that at times I thought he cowered to White men. And it embarrassed me at times. I was also jealous because my friends' fathers were not as strict and I felt like I was missing out. In retrospect, his rearing tactics put me on my current trajectory. I could have easily gone on a much less productive direction and wasted some years, as I have seen in some of my old friends by entering into a life of crime and be swayed by drugs and alcohol. I thought I had a problem with my father and maybe a counselor would have helped me realize that my parents—and my father, in particular—were strict as a demonstration of love and care.

BLACK FATHERING FOR ME NOW

These influences are not just in parenting children in my own home but in supporting young people in my community. My parents have always encouraged me to be a mentor to others, and I know this helped me in my own fathering with my family. My parents' influence on my fathering—no matter who is on the other end of it—is to show love. Sometimes it is tough love, but it still counts as love nonetheless. These were the seeds to how I am fathering my children now; those influences are helping me father Summer Joy and my stepson Justin who has accepted me in to his and his mother's lives. And it hasn't always been easy.

Early on, Ann felt I was trying to buy his affection and that he was at times using me to get video games and other things he wanted. I can admit that it may have been a little of both. I'll have you know that earlier in my life, I vowed never to marry a woman with a child. I was convinced it could be messy and I didn't want to potentially compete with another man as a father figure. And in our case in the earlier years my stepson's biological father was nonexistent.

He warmed quickly. But the one thing I wanted from him—that he still will not give to me—is to call me Dad or some other fatherly name; he adamantly will not.

Perhaps it is a homage to his biological father who has not been as present. I don't know. **But, you should have seen his eyes when he slipped one time and called me "Dad!"** He was so shocked! He has always held steadfast in calling me Kent—and it irks me every time he does it—but he unconsciously loosened up in that moment! Recalling it makes me smile. And I am confident in how I love Justin, no matter what he calls me. He knows my love is unconditional.

In stark contrast, Summer Joy only has eyes for Daddy. Well, not really. She is both a Daddy's Girl and a Mommy's Daughter. Here's what she knows at her age right now; I will give her the world! I think it is partly to honor my mom. I know that if she were living that Summer would not want for anything the same way my mom was with me. When she was just a baby, I wrote the following passage in an effort to capture the moment. I typed it out holding my angel in my arms one evening as she slept. I remember it fondly because I was afraid to put her down. You know how it is when your baby finally falls asleep; I did not want to wake her! And it is these moments that have compelled me to be the father my father was to me, want nothing but the best for my daughter, and doing everything in my power to make sure she gets it!

I wonder what she sees?

After a late night in my office, baby girl was up and at 'em EARLY and with a vengeance! Mommy had her last night. It was my turn. The talkative princess and I ventured downstairs for a little "us" time. She sat in my lap and played and talked and played and talked with her stuffed turtle and praying bear. The moment was endearing, and just then she found her hands. It was as if she had never seen them before; she stared with introspection and continuously put up her index finger. And you know I tried to get a picture, but, hey, my hands were full and the video turned out to be better imagery anyway! At that moment I wondered aloud, "What is it that you see sweetie?" She was definitely into her hands and I was definitely tired, wanting more bed-time as you can tell in the video. But right there, at that moment in time, nothing else mattered.

She was happy! I was in love! And I realized then that my time will always be her time!

We sat until she got restless and decided it was time to walk; sleep was near. We go to the window to look out at the gray and blustery Virginia morning! We stand at the window for what seems like hours. She would look out at the coolness of the brown landscape, and then at me, and then the Christmas tree, back to me again as she periodically grabbed and pulled at my chain. As she pulled looking at me, it was like she was saying with her eyes, "Daddy come closer!" We stand at the window as time passed slowly as I await her sleep. It's uncharacteristically silent; then I fart! My thoughts sprint from, "I wonder what she sees?" to "I wonder what she smells?" We quickly move toward fresher air complimented by the fir scented ornaments as I'm still committed to not put this child down until she is deep into her slumber. These silent and shared moments are golden! I wouldn't trade them for anything in the world!

She sleeps now as I type this, and I wonder no more what she sees. My thoughts revert back to her perfect little fingers; especially the one which positioned itself as to say I am #1. My thoughts immediately turn to the future. My wonder becomes hope, my hope that one day she also will come to know that she is, always has been, and always will be NUMBER ONE! Her Mom and I would have it no other way! Times up! She has now awakened, and I, desperately in LOVE and a little sleep deprived, need to go get her!

Skip to present day

Part of all young children's desire is to feel included, especially when it comes to their daily interactions with the world. Being a part of the fray in many ways helps children to develop a sense of self as they discover themselves in relation to others. This is especially crucial as children start formal schooling, an ideally safe space where children and adolescents develop into social beings. In actuality, these inquiring souls are escorted into institutions that are built on the evaluation of intelligence and conformity all at once. One might find that navigating the educational process to be a daunting task for any young mind still learning their place in the world. History tells us this is especially true for Black students. To this end, it is crucial that we instill three things into our children to help offset the world's cruelty. Black fathers must provide our children with strong mentorship and be role models who empower and provide connection.

Role Modeling and Mentoring. Providing mentoring and role modeling is a way Black fathers can support their own and, when appropriate, others' school-aged children. Effective mentoring provides the nurturing of educational ambitions, develops and increases self-efficacy, and enhances leadership qualities.

Fathers, uniquely positioned, can strategically establish and strengthen mentoring connections between their students, school staff, and community stakeholders.

Student Empowerment Through Father-School Involvement. Black fathers must be involved in the education of their children. They need to have a strong presence within the schools, especially schools whose past and current practices suggest institutionalized racism. To further augment Black students' feelings of belongingness, their fathers must be visible and actively engaged in the education process—ensuring that their children are positively held accountable and understand all possibilities resulting their educational attainments (e.g., leadership opportunities, etc.), especially as they pertain to fair and equitable school policies.

School and Home Connection. Lastly, in an effort to uphold an academic and social sense of belonging, all schools must ensure that meaningful partnerships and opportunities for our involvement are encouraged and maintained. Incorporating Black parents into the school's everyday academic functioning can cultivate a better understanding of race issues and their overall influence on students' educational accomplishments.

The toughest battle

Nothing prepares you for the talk that Black parents have with their children when it comes to their Blackness. We may think we have it all together but what Black father—or any parent—is never ready to hear his child say, "I wish I were White." It sneaks out of the blue, no matter how well we think we've taught them to love themselves. It still happens unexpectedly and it is GUT-WRENCHING! Our thoughts race with questions like:

Is it a stage? How long will it last? How do you replace this unhealthy sense of identity while not stripping your child of their humanity?

And I thought caring for an infant was hard. This is another kind of work—and investment. You actually have to brace yourself to have a difficult conversation with a person who developmentally is not fully capable of understanding what they are experiencing. It is particularly hard when the child is learning the social and academic nuances of school and schooling. What we know is our Black children see the subtle differences in schools themselves in comparison to White and children from other racial and ethnic groups. They see how people respond to the texture of different students' hair when the children are having their hair combed. This happened with my Summer Joy when she brought this up at home. Being the Black father I am, I was determined to make it right for her. I want her to love her skin, her hair, and everything else that makes her uniquely Black. Part of my response was to have my Black female family and friends affirm Summer by helping her see and embrace her own infinite beauty. The Facebook post read:

Summer Joy and Ann! My Pretty Little Black Girls! Shout out to all of my Black Women family and friends! I have an idea and would like to request your assistance! It is my hope to provide my beautiful and intelligent Summer Joy with some positive affirmations that honor Black Womanhood! My Request: Please consider creating a picture of yourself and one of the pictures of Summer Joy attached to this post (unless you actually have a photo with her) that proudly exclaims that "Summer & I are Pretty Black Girls" with a hashtag that represents your skin tone! The skin tone colors that are listed below are examples taken from the children's book "I'm a Pretty Little Black Girl!"; use at your pleasure or add your own special shade! I plan to use your photo to make a collage or album that will serve as a reminder to my baby girl that her Black is truly Beautiful! … and worthy! To all my other friends! If you are so inspired and want to support this effort, please share a quote, affirmation, or an inspired effort from your creative mind that could be included in this project!

Black Girls Rock! #Tan, #Pecan, #Milk in Coffee, #Toffee, #SweetDarkChocolate-Cream, #Cinnamon, #BrownPaperBag, #ButtercupDaisy, #Nutmeg, and a fill in the blank #_____ hashtag, just because. I know I am asking a lot, but I humbly thank you in advance!

The responses poured in and were phenomenal … and therapeutic for my #prettyBlackgirls and me! They really helped to affirm Summer Joy's Blackness. She truly learned to love herself and all her newfound friends who took the time to embrace the agony and pain associated with having to deal with this constant, seemingly never-ending challenge.

This is what Black fathers do; they stand up, and they rise to the occasion. However, it is taxing. I tried to think about how I make it through. In my household, there are two counselors, counselor educators by trade. It should not be this hard, am I right? No, I am not right. When it comes to our Blackness, very little is easy about self-acceptance and others' acceptance. So, where does the strength and resilience come from? What makes it alright? I believe it is my tribe.

My village, my tribe

As a counselor, I believe in the power of counseling. I have definitely sought counseling when needed and sometimes not sought it when I needed it. I have realized that I have not been a client in quite some time, and I am acutely aware of this now. I think the ways I've received a form of counseling support, though, is through my community of counseling friends and colleagues. I am grateful that I'm around counselors on a daily basis. Unbeknownst to them, their insights and expertise are extremely helpful, especially the support I get from my Black male counseling colleagues and friends. We often talk about raising our children and the joys and challenges in it. We find ways to support each other and provide a shoulder to lean on, even unknowingly. Impromptu conversations with them often provide clarity or at least food for thought. Writing this, I marvel at those exchanges because they lift me, and I believe they lift us all!

This oftentimes resulted in a form of counseling support group I did not even know I needed. I am learning as a result that I need my Black counseling brothers in my life. Like my parents, they ground me and remind me I am not alone on the journey of fatherhood. I believe that counselors working with Black fathers during the early childhood education period should embrace this perspective. I strongly encourage and endorse group counseling for Black fathers. There are so many benefits to connecting with people who share a particular challenge or hardship, to find community and get support. I hope Black fathers with experiences similar to mine will not solely rely on men in close proximity (because this is healthy too) but also consider counseling when they want a professional to give them help they can't get from friends and colleagues. And while I did not seek personal counseling about the raising of my daughter, I did seek family counseling services to help me support my stepson which was tremendously useful for us as a family and for me as a father figure to him.

LESSONS LEARNED FROM COUNSELING

Our family counseling helped me to appreciate even more the benefits of counseling. I was reminded that I did not have all of the answers, nor should I expect to have them all. When committed to your children's success, it is probably one of the best things to do, because it allows you to step outside of yourself and see the situation for what it is. You can hear from someone from outside of the experience who has the potential to shed light and reframe situations. Counseling—and the associated work in it—provided opportunities to better understand our challenging circumstances, allowing us to respond to those challenges in healthier ways.

CLOSING THOUGHTS

Every child deserves a chance, especially every Black child! And Black fathers have a role to assume in helping create as many chances as possible. We absolutely need all hands-on deck. It is imperative that outside of the home, Black fathers be advocates for justice and change agents in local schools and communities where they reside. Black fathers are strategically positioned to impact and may positively address the systemic barriers and prejudicial attitudes, behaviors, and practices that hinder our children's development. Black fathers have the potential to proactively impact the lives of many of the students in our children's schools. This being the case, we have an obligation to ensure that our schools provide services that are equitable and uncompromisingly extended to Black students who are often left hanging in the balance awaiting good comprehensive academic and counseling services.

It would behoove counselors and other mental health professionals to genuinely get to know Black fathers and the significance behind relationships with their families. I would encourage counselors to listen to our narratives and the rich stories that govern how they interact and father their children. There is magic in the story. There are lessons and treatment plans in their stories. There is no need to work harder than you need to when, if you let the stories unfold, you have the riches right before you. It is important for counselors to actively listen, engage, and truly enter into the counseling realm with your clients.

As I was finishing the last edits of this chapter, I had another great experience that let me know that I was a very lucky man to be the father of such a wonderful child. As I took a break and was walking to my room to get something, I noticed Summer Joy skipping down the hall to catch up with me. When she reaches me, I ask her if she needed anything as she stood in front of me with her arms and hands straight up past her ears. “No” she says matter-of-factly. “Just a hug.” And just like that, we hugged it out. Parenting is definitely a sacrifice, one that is undeniably worth having. Hands-down, it is absolutely the one thing that I would never trade-in for anything else in the world. The poem below speaks why Black fathers can and must be up to the task when supporting our children within and outside of schools.

I woke myself up
Because we ain’t got an alarm clock
Dug in the dirty clothes basket,
Cause ain’t nobody washed my uniform
Brushed my hair and teeth in the dark,
Cause the lights ain’t on
Even got my baby sister ready,
Cause my mama wasn’t home.
Got us both to school on time,
To eat us a good breakfast.
Then when I got to class the teacher fussed
Cause I ain’t got no pencil

Joshua T. Dickerson

CHAPTER FOUR

Engaged, Non-residential Black Fathering for Early Education Readiness

SAM STEEN, PHD

FATHER PROFILE

Sam Steen is the father of two children and is an associate professor of counseling at George Mason University. Prior to this appointment, Sam worked at The College of William and Mary, George Washington University and the University of Arizona. In addition to a PhD in Education with a specialization in counselor education, Sam is a licensed Professional School Counselor who specializes in school counseling, group work, and students at risk of academic failure. Sam served as a professional school counselor for 10 years prior to entering academia, and his experience as a practitioner heavily shapes his research agenda, approach to teaching, and choices for service. Most recently Sam became Fellow for the Association for Specialists in Group Work (ASGW), a division of the American Counseling Association. Additionally, Sam was the recipient of the Professional Advancement Award for ASGW. This award recognized Sam's outstanding activities in helping advance the field of group work through research, and development of new and innovative strategies for group work in schools and public relations.

INTRODUCTION

This chapter will focus on my experiences as a non-custodial father being intentionally involved in my two children's lives while no longer living in their home. This personal examination includes information that aligns with the research in some cases, but more importantly is an honest account of the balancing act I take when engaging my children in my life. I begin with a summary of my own upbringing including those individuals who were influential in shaping my perspective on fathering. Next, I intersperse what Black fathering looks like for me at this time in my life, in light of the needs of my children and their biracial identity considering their mother is of Filipina descent. I conclude the chapter with a brief summary of my own counseling experiences during a difficult time in life and provide recommendations for counselors who aspire to understand my hopes and struggles as a Black man within this context of fathering children not living within my household.

BIGGEST INFLUENCES ON MY FATHERING

I was raised in a two-parent household that emphasized Christianity. I was raised to have faith in the Bible and to aspire to achieve the best of my abilities. I was also raised to know that others did not determine those abilities. I heard specific messages, "No matter how much talent, intelligence or skills in school or sports you have, it will be necessary to be diligent in your endeavors in order to reach your fullest potential." While I was raised with both of my parents in my household, these lessons came from my father and mother at different times. At other times these messages came from my extended biological and community family; they were my aunts, uncles, older brother, teachers, pastors, basketball coaches, and friends.

These messages from my family and community made me feel that I could accomplish anything and that I could be both confident in my skills and also to help others achieve their dreams. I truly believed this because I saw my father in particular set all types of goals and accomplish them while also encouraging others to do the same. The types of things I recall include military ranks and promotions, competition within intramural sports, taking speaking lessons, and engaging in debates with toast masters and also chess. As a consequence, when I envisioned being a father I assumed it would be an easy feat and that the woman I marry will help me with this process. I also believed that fathers are the breadwinners and responsible for teaching children how to play sports.

Over time, even as a non-residential father, these enduring messages both resonate and inform how I father my children. I currently reside in a different home than my two children who live with their biological mother. My daughter is 13 years old and my son is eight years old. I moved from their house three years ago, so for a portion of their lives I lived with them. During those years in their home, there was a lot of strife and turmoil interspersed with love, kindness, and affection. The current living arrangements mean that the components of their family of origin went from mom, dad, and children to divorced parents, single mom household, and dad with a new wife of less than one year. Put another way, their mother and I went from focusing on our relationship as husband and wife to shift squarely on them, their perspective of this world, their feelings, thoughts, hopes, and dreams as mutually involved and concerned parents.

BLACK FATHERING FROM A NON-CUSTODIAL PERSPECTIVE

Birth

When my daughter was born, I was in the middle of completing my dissertation. The obstetrician told us she would be born in late August and I was determined to finish by August 10. I thought this would give us a few weeks to just revel in what was about to drastically change in my life all around me. I worked diligently to meet my August 10 deadline. When August 10 came, I was not finished. But guess who arrived?! My daughter was born on August 10 at 7PM! I learned very quickly that infants do a lot of eating, sleeping, and moving their bowels.

Thankfully, my parental leave benefits allowed me to complete my dissertation—with all the necessary edits and revisions—and defend in November before returning back to work. Her birth helped focus me in a way that I had not recalled in my life up to that point. I genuinely believed that I was the happiest man alive.

And while the dynamic between her mother and I was not perfect, I made a commitment to focus on doing whatever I could to keep the household balanced and full of love. Soon after her birth, I transitioned into an academic position. You have to understand; I was a first-generation college graduate, now with a PhD and job as a professor. One privilege from earning the doctorate was that my position at the time afforded me the opportunity to stay home beginning in January when she was approximately a year and a half.

I was a stay-at-home dad for the better part of eight months between January and August. I am certain that this was a first in my family.

Stereotypically, Black fathers are described as absent in their young children's lives or less involved. I was determined to challenge this narrative. During this time, my daughter and I would attend all sorts of events together. We would do "mommy and me" events at the library and local shopping centers, even when

I was the only parent who wasn't a mommy. We would go to parks and spend time with neighbors who were also stay-at-home parents. During this time, I was becoming painfully aware that I would be one of the few—if not the sole—fathers present at these events, but that came with the territory. I was proud and grateful to have the time and resources to do what I was doing in these early years.

Unfortunately, there were some tensions that emerged as her mother and I worked through co-parenting. Simply put, her mom didn't like how I interacted with our daughter. She was determined that I should raise her like a little girl and not a little boy. She was basically implying that I was too rough and I did not use soft language when communicating with her. In fact, she also mentioned that sometimes I was raising her to be less sophisticated than she would have liked. It was hard to hear this, honestly. I couldn't help but assume that her comments were because I'm Black. This wasn't the first time I heard the same type of comments or sentiment during our relationship. The language in her assertions were subtly coded in racial and gendered ways. I was able to remind her mother that my role as a father was to be a dad, and for me that meant using language was most natural to me to ensure that I was being genuine. I was not interested in being someone I'm not and then have to keep up a farce in order to communicate with her as she aged.

To this day my daughter and I have a great relationship due to this time-intensive foundation that was started when she was really young.

I do suspect that some of the challenges between my daughter's mom and me were related to my flexible work schedule. It must have been tough for her to see me stay home and spend so much quality time with her while she had to go to work.

Five years later our son was born. However, prior to his birth, I already decided that I needed to leave the relationship and household because there was too much tension and conflict between us to remain. I did not feel like myself. In fact, I have vivid memories of looking into the mirror often, painfully reconciling that I did not want to live like this for the rest of my life. I made the hard decision. Four months before he was born I moved out of my home and with my uncle. As irony would have it—while at a New Year's Eve party—my wife called me to let me know she might be in labor. I immediately left to meet her and our daughter at the hospital. I am grateful that I made it to witness his arrival on January 1! What a lucky and blessed baby to be born on a day when people across the country (and world) will be celebrating each year for the rest of his life!

Naturally, there was a lot taking place that day and during that time for me and for my family. But personally, I would say that the second most important thing that happened that day was a conversation—if that's what you would call it—between my younger sister and me.

That morning, she called and firmly told me that it was necessary for me to take my Black ass home. She said that it was not the little man's fault that there was tension between his parents, and that it would be necessary to try and establish a firm foundation for him, like we had done for his sister and like my parents had done for me.

I listened. I honestly tried to make it work. I moved back in and stayed for about three years. Unfortunately, I was only able to cope with the strife in our household by avoiding intense contact and emotional involvement with my wife. In fact, we abstained from sexual contact for the duration of this time. Was this helpful? Did this actually work? I am not sure. But I am sure of my effort and work to spend as much time with him as possible and to be intentional about developing a relationship with him. What I did not anticipate was that I would end up moving across the country when he turned five.

Gender

Collectively, we are raising two children. But, I often refer to them as a young woman and young man intentionally to sadly remind them that they will be perceived outwardly as a Black woman and Black man in our community as people of color. Children of color, including Black children, are stereotyped and perceived often as older in a range of social settings. Even with that I was always intentional in my engagement with both of my children. I would teach my daughter different outdoor games and sports, sometimes engaging in what might be considered rough and tumble play. Thankfully, I learned over time she was much more appreciative of activities that were not as physical or competitive. With my son, I was more physically and emotionally absent as he was growing up. When we did spend time together, I would take him running, doing outdoor activities like looking for bugs, and playing various sports. I also made a concerted effort with teaching them both how to cook, to help build their confidence and comfort in the kitchen.

But gender dynamics has been a struggle at times, and even now. I struggled with the language I would use with my children. Here's one example. I would sometimes call my daughter "little man", just because I thought it was cute. This was not received well by her mother. I mean, not at all. And although I was resistant to stopping it because of her mother's preference, I stopped. Her mom suggested that it might cause identity confusion for our daughter. And this is another layer of difficulty for me. I recognize I can and have embraced gender stereotypes and mistruths. Here is how I know.

I have been more intentional at making sure I was treating my son as a boy, little man, and now growing young man because I have feared that maybe my son would be more effeminate because I did not live with him.

And my fears were exacerbated when—at times—he wanted to dress like his mother and sister. I would not necessarily discourage him outwardly when this happened. However, I would make it very clear that it was not funny or cute like his mother or sister thought. I do not have those fears now but when he was younger—and I was younger, less mature, and more frequently absent—I struggled with these types of incidences and my feelings associated with them. I felt guilty that I was not living in the household fulltime and falsely assumed that the amount of time he was spending with women and girls only was because of my less than consistent presence. What has helped my growth in this area is my professional counseling community and role as a professor. I have been challenged by faculty, staff, and students to use non-gender conforming language when referring to the class (e.g., greeting with "good evening folks" versus "good evening, ladies and gentlemen"). This indeed was a learning curve for me. Around this time our local K-12 public schools started to offer non-gender conforming bathrooms and this encouraged my intentional efforts at using verbal language and body language that was consistent with being less rigid and judgmental. I still have a way to go in this area, but living closer to my children and taking time to ask them questions makes me feel better. It means that I have an opportunity to model for them what is more aligned with my own upbringing and my desires for them as they navigate our changing world. These messages were important to me as a young Black man growing up, and I'm integrating appropriate messages that align with my values and desires for our children.

As you can imagine, fathering while not living with my children means trying to help them make sense of the world—and its complex issues—without me being immediately present. These are just a few more examples that have been particularly salient.

Race and racism

My children go to predominantly white schools, and they are becoming more and more aware of their racial identities. They have Black and Filipino/a heritage; they are Black and their skin is fairer than mine, but they do not look white. I know, though, they have heard and internalized racist messages. One discussion I had with my 13-year-old daughter made me aware that she refers to herself with her white friends as a "brownie." At first, I was adamant that was not the most accurate way to identify in relation to whiteness and white people. I learned, though, that at least one of her white friends mentioned that this was inappropriate too. I also had to reconcile that this was not about me and that I was not in her skin. She was learning to identify in ways she wanted, and possibly needed. I learned over time that she was comfortable with sharing how salient her beautiful, brown, sweet skin was with her friends and some of them were uncomfortable pointing out those differences.

School involvement

One of the most challenging aspects of being a non-custodial father is consistent school involvement. Deciding who is responsible for attending Back to School Nights, open houses, parent–teacher conferences, and so on is an ongoing discussion. This is challenging and must be negotiated up front if the children's custodial roles are up for negotiation. Research continues to demonstrate that school involvement by parents and families has a direct positive correlation to student achievement (Griffin & Steen, 2010). Building and sustaining school parent and community involvement for Black and other families of color is often considered more difficult to accomplish (Bryan & Henry, 2012; Hannon, 2020). Who is responsible for making the effort to get more families involved? There are a number of barriers to parental involvement including scheduling conflicts, personal feelings about one's own early school experiences, school demographics, and the school's administration, faculty, and staff's ability to embrace multiculturalism in schools (Epstein et al., 2019). Along those lines, fathers are often targeted by schools who desire more involvement by dads in order to help them feel welcomed.

One really interesting program that I participate in on a regular basis at my son's elementary school is called "WatchDOGS." More specifically, Dads of Great Students is a program designed squarely to get fathers involved.

This program does not target Black fathers in particular, but it does make it really clear what the expectations are for dads who are able to spend an entire day at their child's school as the fathers will be involved in most aspects of the school day.

These activities include helping with drop off in the morning, doing classroom activities, helping with cafeteria duty, and other important activities on any given school day. This program from personal experience is wonderful. The structure it provides allows for dads to get involved quickly and to know exactly what to do and when. But the personal challenges I've experienced when volunteering at my son's school involve cultural mismatches. Black students are still suffering from numerous stereotypes when it comes to schooling in general and academic achievement in particular (DeBell, 2008). I personally can say I have suffered from stereotype threat (Steele & Aronson, 1995), or the idea that if the school personnel with whom I am interacting believe that I have deficits then I'll either confirm those deficits or present in a way that is less helpful at me being able to dispel those assumptions. This is despite my advanced degrees, background in school counseling, and scholarly accomplishments. At the same time, the potential value added for Black men being present in the school stands to benefit the entire school community because it can begin to dispel racial stereotypes and normalize Black male presence.

For the past two years I have spent one full day at his school each month. Regardless of this consistent involvement I have felt pressure. The purpose for me getting involved so intentionally is to provide an opportunity for my son—and other children, faculty, and staff by proxy—to see me in school and hopefully offset stereotypes associated with parents of color including the faulty narrative that many lack willingness to be involved in their child's school.

Family planning

Conflict in relationships is unavoidable, but can be necessary. Some conflict creates opportunities for people to honestly voice their opinions and feelings. I have learned that conflict can be uncomfortable, but conflict avoidance can be damaging. At one point in my marriage to my children's mother, I became conflict avoidant, and at that point I knew the relationship would not recover. I am grateful, though, that the ending of our marriage has, over time, created a more collaborative relationship which benefits our children. I am especially aware of this as a noncustodial parent who is in a new, married relationship. I consistently think about the role my wife has in my children's lives. I also wonder about my own family planning now.

My wife and I do not have children together yet, but I suspect if/when we do everyone in our extended family system will need time, space, and understanding to adjust to a new dynamic. I have taken time to ask my daughter and son how they would feel if we have more children. They both assure me that this would be fine. My son has told me that he likes being the youngest because he has a lot of people to take care of him. He is aware that with a new sibling he may be responsible for taking care of someone else. I am grateful he has shared this perspective with me.

I am especially sensitive about tensions that might develop between my former wife, my current wife, and my children's visitations. I am grateful there have not been any challenges but I know issues like disciplining can be touchy. My current wife and I have talked intentionally about how she is free to give me feedback on disciplining my children and I welcome that feedback. I believe this will help in a few ways. First, this will present her as an active member of our family and can reinforce messages their mother and I communicate to the children. It can also help augment the work I am doing with them as a father. As my partner, my current wife and I can support each other by providing my children with a bonus caretaker and a loving adult in their lives. And I love the prospect of this.

Finances

I've learned a lot about managing finances in the last several years and I wish my parents were more intentional about teaching me about finances earlier in my life. It has taken me about 19 years to get out of debt from student/college loans, credit card(s) that I got in my very first semester in college. It is only now—in large part with the support from my wife's knowledge of finance—that I and we save and invest money in a variety of ways. I now plan to discuss and teach sound money management with my children to help them understand the difference between earning money and spending money.

I've learned that debt was a form of incarceration for me because it limited my freedom to do what I believe was reasonable as a fully employed, highly educated and responsible Black man.

I realize that as their noncustodial father there will be differences in how their mother and I discuss money with them and our influence on them is still to be determined. I believe teaching my children how to be responsible with their money is even more salient for them as people of color to assist them in attaining financial stability and even wealth.

Spirituality

It's important for me to say that I am a Christian man. I do my best to model what it means to be a follower of Jesus Christ. Two important parts of my Christian journey and identity are prayer and attending a local church. My kids and I pray together when we first get in the car, when picking them up to come and visit with me. I also pray on their behalf with them when I bring them back to their home. When we eat each meal together, I ask them to take turns offering the blessing over the food. In addition to prayer, I try to model with my language how important the Lord has been in our family despite the challenges associated with my marriage to their mother, the loss of three of four of their grandparents, challenges going on around them in the media, or things they hear about in school. We have not found a church that we attend regularly in this new community where I live, but it is something that will undoubtedly happen in the next couple of years as these things take time from my experience.

INTENTIONAL ENGAGEMENT AS A NON-CUSTODIAL BLACK FATHER

The strategies I use to engage my children include prayer primarily and open communication on all things. When I pray aloud and sometimes ask them to do the same, it is an opportunity for me to be vulnerable to them because it allows them to hear what's on my heart. I do not do it for show; I do it to share my deepest thoughts, feelings, and aspirations, even if only for a brief moment.

Another strategy I use when we spend time together—in person or from a distance—is to ask them for daily or weekend reflections. This includes sharing with me something that really stood out to them that was positive, and something that might have been less positive.

The purpose of these discussions is to capitalize, even in small ways, the experiences that they may have had during what might seem like random events to them, but what are really intentional experiences facilitated by me.

I allow them to pick from a few choices, and I try really hard to not make it seem like every time they are with me equates to vacation or endless amounts of fun. This could pose an unrealistic expectation, and I would never want for them to compare their time with me with their time with their mother in unhealthy ways.

One intentional way I connected with my daughter was just a few years ago. When she was around 12, I lived in a different state from her and her brother. It was during this time that we developed a daily check-in routine before she got on the bus for school. It was brief; only five or six minutes at a time. But, it was invaluable. And, in all honesty, it was difficult given the time zone difference between us. I was on west coast time and she was on east coast time. A 7:45AM call for her meant a 4:45AM call for me. Often during these calls I would pray for her and sometimes would ask her to pray for us. Every so often she would refuse and I never made a fuss as I believe prayer is something that should be optional and not forced. We did this her entire 7th grade year with merely missing only three or four times due to sickness or if she was running late. I would still travel to see her and her brother every month for about five days at a time, and during these visits I could clearly see that our relationship had deepened from the ongoing connection that occurred while I was away.

Another strategy I use to engage with them is to volunteer at their school. These volunteer opportunities are not always squarely centered on their specific classroom—meaning I may not volunteer to read in my 3rd grader's class, but I may come and help out in the library or during a book fair, or even during field day. For the middle school I have taken a more passive approach and tried to help with administrative tasks for the School Counseling department as these activities align with my professional background, interests, and skillset. I also try to attend the Parent Teacher Association (PTA) meetings and also help with picture day which in no way is a prestigious job.

These strategies mentioned above are used to create and sustain an emotional (e.g., through prayer) as well as a physical connection (e.g., visibility in school) with my children. I enjoy schools because of my career as an educator, but I also enjoy extracurricular activities.

I spend time with my children sporadically but primarily on the weekends, holidays, and during extensive periods in the summer. This loose schedule developed when I lived 3500 miles away for nearly three years. I have since moved back and live only 19 miles away from them now. But what I have found is that I must remain intentional about the timing of our visits, the goals for our interactions (unbeknownst to them), and providing room for them to reflect on our time together.

COUNSELING SUPPORT I NEEDED TO NAVIGATE THIS EXPERIENCE

Raising children and adolescents who are not living in your household presents a number of considerations as mentioned. These include logistical things like scheduling. But they also include considerations like fostering healthy identity development, developing open communication pathways, decisions about discipline methods, and the list goes on. I've navigated these barriers over the past few years and believe that I have gained the following insights that could be useful for counseling professionals.

First, counselors working with Black non-residential fathers should remember that we all need a supportive network comprised of close friends, family members, clergy, or even neighbors. Counselors can help the fathers assess who is in their support network and determine how accessible they are for them. Regardless of who we rely on for support, it is imperative that we seek ongoing assistance when necessary and counselors can and should inquire about this with their clients.

I actually tried to take advantage of counseling support, specifically marriage counseling, prior to my son being born. Unfortunately, the counselor I sought was not very skilled in helping me with my presenting problem which essentially was helping me to find ways to reduce the strife and conflict between my children's mother and me. Specifically, at the conclusion of one of our counseling sessions, I shared deeply with my therapist a desire for her to be more transparent with me. I desired self-disclosure from her with regard to the external stressors (e.g., pressure to succeed, fear of failure, oppression, marginalization, stereotype threat) I experienced as a Black man that might impact the internal deficits I was experiencing. Quite frankly, I let her know that I was a counselor educator and was currently teaching a supervision course for therapists in training. Additionally, I asked her if she was open to receiving some suggestions and feedback on my experiences with her to date. She obliged and below I will provide a snapshot of what I suggested to her, along with a few others that I have gleaned from my scholarly pursuits. In retrospect I wonder if my role as an instructor stood in the way of role as a client. I'm not sure I'll ever know, but I have learned a lot and that I hope counselors can use from my experience.

Counselors can encourage Black fathers to be intentional about capitalizing on simple moments they have with their children, regardless of where they live. Parenting is arduous, no doubt. And being a non-residential father can be a huge barrier to making important connections to children. But being a Black father is also deeply rewarding. If a father has had great experiences as a child and great role models for fatherhood, then the choices to stay involved are likely inherent. If a father has not had this privilege during their upbringing, then there may be more explicit challenges such as how vulnerable to be with their children while attempting to remain strong and courageous in everyday life. To this point, as counselors work with Black non-custodial fathers and gain more knowledge through the assessing and exploration they can learn what their Black father clients have seen and been taught about fatherhood. It likely influences how they will father. I also cannot underscore the value of counselors validating Black fathers' experiences in therapeutic care as African Americans get sicker and die more often from preventable and treatable illnesses than any other racial group (Edwards & Erwin-Johnson, 2003). Some of this requires their Blackness to be acknowledged and affirmed.

The skill of broaching is critical in working with clients, particularly when it comes to issues of race and other identities. I say address it, and address it openly. Please look me—and other Black fathers in therapy—in the eyes and see us as we are. Please do not discount our feelings when we rant about how emotionally draining it can be when we see racist stereotypes about Black men reinforced in the media that we are violent, scary, devious, ignorant, do not belong, or are up to no good.

Please let us share this. Please help us express the anger, fear, resentment, fatigue, and pain that our community continues to experience. Please listen with a non-judgmental and open stance.

Second, I would urge counselors to please acknowledge that past and present encounters with racism, oppression, and microaggressions are real, even if they cannot relate. Historical trauma is defined as the cumulative emotional and psychological wounding over one's life, and across generations stemming from massive group trauma scenarios (Brave Heart, 2003). It is real and impacts Black people in contemporary society. Enduring chronic discrimination is related to higher allostatic load—which essentially translates into high blood pressure, high cortisol levels, increased heart rates, and can result it depression, anxiety, and other mental health issues. (Ong, Williams, Nwizu & Gruenewald, 2017).

Third, counselors must continue to be strength-based in their orientation and treatment methods. I realize that honesty about what I might be experiencing—even if incredibly hard—might be exactly what I need to be hopeful and persist when in the face of obstacles that exist as a result of racism. Helping Black fathers discover, or rediscover, their strengths by confirming the resilience necessary to overcome the insidious nature of racism and oppression may give us the unconditional positive regard, and therapeutic breakthrough necessary to be the best fathers we can be as Black men. While the non-custodial situation might not be ideal, an effective counseling relationship is potentially sufficient enough to augment the relationships being established within the family. Finally, I would ask counselors to consider reminding Black fathers that life is precious and life is short. I say precious because moment by moment is not promised, and short, because I personally lost my father to prostate cancer when he was 65 years old. My dad was 23 years old when I was born and died when I turned 42. I am 45 years old and determined to be the best father I can be, and I hope that sharing my personal experiences can in some way be helpful for therapists who desire to help other Black fathers face these challenges I have described.

REFERENCES

Brave Heart, M. Y. (2003). The historical trauma response among natives and its relationship with substance abuse: A Lakota illustration. *Journal of Psychoactive Drugs*, *35*, 7–13.

Bryan, J. & Henry, L. (2012). A model for building school-family-community partnerships: Principles and process. *Journal of Counseling and Development, 90* (4), 408–420. https://doi.org/10.1002/j.1556-6676.2012.00052.x

DeBell, M. (2008). Children living without their fathers: Population estimates and indicators of educational well-being. *Social Indicators Research, 87*(3), 427–443. https://doi.org/10.1007/s11205-007-9149-8

Epstein, J. L., et al. (2019). *School, Family, and Community Partnerships: Your Handbook for Action*. Fourth edition. Thousand Oaks, CA: Corwin Press.

Hannon, L. V. (2020). *You don't know my story: Engaging Black parents with culturally responsive school practices*. Doctoral dissertation, Montclair State University.

Steele, C. M., & Aronson, J. (1995). Stereotype threat and the intellectual test performance of African-Americans. *Journal of Personality and Social Psychology*, *69*, 797–811.

Griffin, D., & Steen, S. (2010). School-Family-Community Partnerships: Applying Epstein's Theory of the Six Types of Involvement to School Counselor Practice. *Professional School Counseling, 13, 218–226*. DOI.org/10.5330/PSC.n.2010-13.218

Edwards, W. V., & Erwin-Johnson, C. (2003). NAACP to focus on minority health disparities. *Crisis (The New)*, *110*, 54—56.

Ong, A. D., Williams, D. R., Nwizu, U., & Gruenewald, T. L. (2017). Everyday unfair treatment and multisystem biological dysregulation in African-American Adults. *Cultural Diversity & Ethnic Minority Psychology*, *23*, 27—35.

CHAPTER FIVE

Fathering Biracial Children in the 21st Century

LINWOOD G. VEREEN, PHD

FATHER PROFILE

I am a 51-year-old, heterosexual, cisgender, Black man who has fathered five children who are all biracial. I am partnered with a woman who fully supports me in my role as a father while also challenging me to be my best self as a human being. In my current loving relationship, I am reminded by my partner that not only do my children need me as a constant in their life in the present moment but also that in their future as young adults they will, as a way of making sense of the world, require different levels of support and nurturance from me as their father. My hope is that my children and I have developed a set of relationships that will allow that to occur but at the same time know that this is not the case for all of them. I say that it is my hope because I have for the last decade been estranged from my oldest child, and this has had a profound impact on my fathering profile and my daily existence. It has in my mind and heart left a void not only for me but also for my four other children. My younger four children know of their older sister and have heard many stories about her as a child, teenager, and then as a younger adult. Here is where the stories end due to a lack of contact and connection. My children are four young women and one young man who range in age from 35 to 3. Fathering is an important part of my identity and for longer that I can remember has been an integral part of my identity. It also serves as a critical lens through which I view the world and answer complex questions such as how do

I reconcile violent messages toward women in music as the father of four women? How do I raise my son to honor women as dynamic beings and simultaneously avoid becoming a target of police violence and brutality? How can I raise him to be an advocate, ally, and social accomplice to women, boys, men, same gender loving persons, transgender persons, and all humans in our spectrum? I realize that as a part of my fathering profile I would like to raise the world to not see my son as a threat. I am unfortunately powerless to raise the world. I can, however, influence the world through how I raise my children and, in turn, how they as my children raise me to be a productive father who takes on multiple perspectives and is open to learning with and from them. I hope that as a part of my fathering profile that I will someday be the father for them that they have both dreamed of and they have enjoyed value their journey through youth and adulthood. I am raising biracial children, and I realize that first and foremost the world continues to see, assess, and judge them as Black. My profile as a father began at the age of 16 and as one could imagine I was ill prepared for the role. I hope that at the age of 51 as I write these words I have grown as a father and am well on my journey to being my best self as a father. Raising biracial and multiracial children is difficult when the world only sees them as being Black and exotic, having good hair or not, or as being able to walk between multiple spaces and realities. My truth of the matter is simple. Although they are biracial, my children are seen in the world as being Black. How is it that I then raise them to embrace their Blackness as beautiful and also honor their Puerto Rican and white heritage in meaningful ways that fuel their soul? This is my journey as a father.

BIGGEST INFLUENCES ON MY FATHERING

I have been fortunate to have many important fathering influences in my life. My influences as a father comprise both who (i.e., people) and what (i.e., experiences). The who are a list of people who I have had the privilege, joy, and sometimes heartache to live with, learn from, grow with, and cry and laugh with. The what represents the experiences with a list of profound women, men, and children who have and continue to influence me as a person, human being, and father. My aim here is to present them in a manner so you can feel the impact of them on me as I walk my existential path as a father in current society.

My first fathering influence was and remains my mother who was born Willie Mae Hopkins. For much of the 1970s when she unceremoniously began her role as a single parent following the split from my father Stacey through 2009 when she died and to this day still, she serves as my most profound influence as a father. She is my "who's who" among those who have influenced me as a person and father. She raised seven children as a single mother and taught me things that no other human being could quite accomplish. Although she has been dead for over 10 years at this point, her impact on me is eternal. As a young man I have no recollection of my mother ever telling me, "No you can't do that." The absence of these words in my memory are profound because she at the same time was telling me, "You can do anything." I'm certain that over the course of my life that my mother told me that it was not in my best interest to engage in certain behaviors yet I have no vivid memory of her saying no to anything other than she was strongly against my desire to get married at the tender age of 19.

When I walked into the house with my newborn daughter at the age of 16 to change her diaper, my mother had a range of choices and decisions that she could have exercised in that moment.

What she chose to do was to show me how to properly change a diaper and how to hold her like a baby and not a football. She chose to not scream at me, she chose to not belittle me, but instead loved me through this time in my life which left an indelible influence on me that to this day impacts how I interact with my children. The message that I received from my mother and all of my subsequent influences on my fathering was first to attend to the human aspect of "being in the world" and then to all other issues and concerns. The most important thing about fathering is to be present and an active being in each moment with your child. This can be an amazingly difficult task at any moment in time but at the same time provides a joy in my life that can't be quantified.

As a 12-year-old "Pop Warner football star" I made what turned out to be a poor choice. I once played a bad game and attributed it to the fact that my mother was present at the game. I was ridiculously superstitious and recalled that I never played poorly when she wasn't in attendance, so the reason I was awful had to be because she was there. I mustered the courage to ask her to stop attending my games, and she reluctantly complied with my wish. Imagine the absurdity I feel today about this story. As I later excelled as a high school athlete in track, football, and for a hot minute basketball, I did it in isolation. As my friends and peers left the court or field they walked to their family and to their parents while I walked in solitude to the locker room for four years of high school. I realize how lonely that walk was and how I don't want that sense of loneliness and isolation for my children. At the conclusion of my senior year of high school, I was invited to participate in an All-Star football game with some of my home state's brightest and best athletes. For a short time, I felt as if I didn't belong on the same field as this group of young men. I felt an overwhelming sense of being an imposter and that I would soon be exposed. This changed for me when I became angry at myself for doubting myself. I would love for my children to never doubt themselves, yet if this happens I would also want for them to become angry for doubting their place in this world. This is a challenge that still occurs for me, and that is often times mitigated and disrupted by the fearlessness that I see in my children when they engage in their activities of choice or are simply enjoying the challenge of the local playground. After getting over myself, I played with a reckless abandon and a freedom that made the game fun for me and crushed my fears. I was at the end of it all—humbled and sobbing—when at the end of the game as I was taking my ritual lonely walk to the locker room I was confronted with the sight of my mother. I did a double take to try to convince my mind and my heart that I wasn't dreaming and that she was really there. And, yes, she was.

What I have learned from that experience is that even though not always present, she is always there, she is always with me, and more importantly for my soul, that she has always been there.

Seeing my mother at that moment affirms for me today that my children, much like me, want to know that I am there, that I am present, and that I see them. I see them as beautiful people who have multiple identities and who while the world sees them as Black, they are biracial. While it has been difficult due to divorce and the blending of families, many years later, my children know and seem to fully believe that I am with them always even when I am not physically present. They know that I will always come for them when they need me the most and when they expect it the least. This is the influence of Willie Mae. This is fathering.

My brief period as a Pop Warner football star was guided by Mr. Miller. I don't know that I ever knew his first name but I remember and feel the impact that he had on me as a person and as a result, on my fathering. Mr. Miller always told me the simple truth. I wish I could say with conviction that I live that way always but I am learning as I walk my fathering journey. Mr. Miller placed me at right guard on offense because that is what he felt was needed for our team to succeed. Keep in mind that at this time in my life I was 130 pounds of me. I was angry and played that way. I guess that made Mr. Miller look like he knew what he was doing as a coach. In the middle of our first game, Mr. Miller changed his mind about how I could best help the team. He moved me to play running back. While I was relieved to move into a skill position I still wanted to be the quarterback. I wanted to be like Doug Williams or any star Black quarterback in college at that time. What Mr. Miller taught me was honesty in the face of tough choices, patience, service to others, and commitment. My commitment to my team was bigger than me. As a father, my commitment to my children is bigger than me. I believe in service and try to help my children see value in service, the virtue of honesty, and patience with themselves as they grow into their way of being in this world.

These traits were further developed when I arrived at college. Brian Usher was my coach then and is a friend now; he has nurtured me in ways that he doesn't even realize that influence how I am with my children. His children were fixtures at our football practices so I watched him love and nurture them while at the same time being firm and fair. I noticed that he was this way with everyone. He has always been firm, fair, consistent, loving, and caring. In the over 35 years that I have known this man he is always the same. I want for my children to feel consistent love and care with me. Steve Spagnuola is another of my college coaches who has been an influence on my fathering which is profound for me since he has no children of his own. I learned from him the value of persistence, and the importance of providing motivation and supporting that motivation through consistent encouragement. To this day he states "iron sharpens iron" and the meaning I take from this quote is that the strength and nurturing that I give my children allows them the capacity to be strong and own that part of themselves. I want for my children to live a fearless life and know their inner strength.

From my mother and Charlie Adams who mentored me at my neighborhood Boys Club … Wait, let me offer many thanks to all who worked and raised resilient young men and women at the Jerome Orcutt Boys' and Girls' Club … I learned patience, dignity, and hard work. To raise seven children or to coordinate a Boys' and Girls' Club in a city neighborhood coping with disinvestment takes a great deal of patience. I feel that witnessing these traits allow me to be a patient listener for my children and a nurturing parent. This in turn helps me see them as diverse individuals in a world that can't wait to judge and label them. Charlie Adams is a man who came into my life at a time when I was in need of direction and perspective.

From Charlie Adams I received guidance, patience, and was able to bear witness to a living example of a man who seemed to flawlessly balance the joy of fatherhood with the mission of engaging in otherfathering to raise Black boys into their adulthood.

This man came into my life and showed me that it was not ok to hit, yell, resort to violence, or demean another human being. He showed me through examples how love, patience, and listening to hear and learn could empower a struggling Black boy to be his best self. Through my experiences with this man I now know that I learned through action. I will initially tell anyone who will listen that at this time in my life I learned how to swim, play basketball, shoot pool, and engage in sports with a healthy sense of intensity and fear that drove me to excel. What I often times overlook is how at this point in my life and existence I learned patience, vulnerability, how to listen, how to engage in conflict resolution, how to love, and how to express that love in healthy ways in my youth from Charlie Adams. These empowering experiences were consistently in conflict with alternate experiences, stereotypes, and fears that led me to treat people poorly at times and live up to the negative perceptions of what it meant to be a Black boy in an inner city. I experienced an inner conflict that I want to shield from my children. I want them to live one life, one existence, and to live it fully and unapologetically in full view of the world. I hope that they never live in a duality of existence, yet at the same time I realize that this occurs consistently for Black girls and Black boys who grow to be Black women and Black men. In my heart I feel that the challenge is alternately different for biracial children. My fathering work is to help them grow to love themselves as whole people and honor all of who they are. I hope that they remember and never forget that they are Black and at the same time are white and Puerto Rican.

My other and equally profound fathering influences were athletic coaches Desmond Robinson (college football), Bill Chagnon (freshman high school basketball), and Frank Savo Jr. (high school football). These men showed me love, kindness, were patient, encouraging, and consistently evidenced a belief in my ability to be successful in the areas of my choice. Additionally, these men would not allow me to leave and behave in ways that they felt were embarrassing to me or my family. Each—in their own way—instilled in me a desire to define for myself and then seek to achieve goals that would benefit my life circumstance. Desmond Robinson affirmed my fathering belief in "showing up." As he recruited me to play football, he showed me that I was more than a prospective student athlete; he showed me that I mattered as a young Black man and that I had a rightful place in this world. In my mind, I feel he was always looking after me and wanting more for me than to be a football player. In my heart I felt as if this Black man who was not my father was happy to be my otherfather. When he left the University of Connecticut after my first year for a better coaching opportunity, he continued to show up by reaching out to me to check on me through direct contact and through contact with the other coaches in the football team. He is but one on a list of remarkable people who fathered me and loved me unconditionally. When I told him that I was thinking of leaving school because I was not earning an opportunity to play and had to redshirt, he confronted me for not trusting in our relationship to confide in him my thoughts and feelings.

I saw in this moment a man who was not afraid of losing a recruit but a man, who as my otherfather, was afraid of losing me to the streets of Bridgeport, Connecticut.

I saw a man who realized that if I left, the chances were dramatically high that I would not find another institution of higher education to attend. He was afraid that I would not earn a degree, thus further increasing my chances of becoming a negative statistic. Desmond Robinson took up after Frank Savo, Jr. the role of being my otherfather when I left high school. He took on this role as I was still in high school and held that role for some years. Frank Savo, Jr. as my otherfather transformed my life by asking me one simple question. He asked me, "Would you go to college if I could help get you in?" This simple question altered my life trajectory because prior to this I had planned to join the Army after high school. I had planned to travel the world in service to my country and be a global citizen and protector of a nation and its citizens, who consistently fail to protect me and people who look like me. Suddenly, the world opened up for me, and there was now newfound potential and opportunity. A loving and caring white man joined in the community of people who raised me to open doors to access and opportunity. He taught me through and about the subject of high school football. While he fostered my growth to excel as an athlete, he more importantly fostered my growth as human being and influenced how I am with my own children. He always showed up. While I foster the growth of my children in their pursuits of choice and other critical areas of life, I more importantly father their growth as dynamic human beings who are capable of great things. This is what Frank Savo Jr. did for me as my otherfather. In otherfathering me he took the mantle from Bill Chagnon who I think both knew and didn't know the impact of his otherfathering on me. He also had no way of knowing that how he helped to raise a 14 year-old Black boy would help him grow to thrive as a Black man.

One day while playing in a freshman high basketball game that was nearly over—and we were winning—I began to taunt players from the opposing team. With less than two minutes left in the game, my coach Bill Chagnon called timeout, removed me from the game, and promptly and quietly pulled me aside to inform me that my behavior was embarrassing to myself, my family, and my team. He confronted me in such a caring way that I did not feel embarrassed and I was able to hear in that moment, without reservation, his care, thoughts, and concerns. He, much like my mother, called me out in a manner that affirmed my dignity and humanity while at the same time let me know that in no uncertain terms my behavior was not fitting of who I was and who I was to become. These are but a few examples of the influence that I have been privileged to experience that have positively impacted my fathering.

Without question, the biggest influence on my fathering comes from my children. They provide for me a constant source of love, care, and support. They instill in me the capacity for silly behavior, making messes while cooking, random dance parties, "monfer (i.e., monster) tag," and movie night with homemade caramel popcorn.

I often state that my children are raising me to be a good father.

I believe that their influence on me lies in the reciprocal nature of our relationship. Developmentally, my younger children are unaware that we are engaged in a reciprocal relationship that is grounded in love, trust, and admiration for the other. They are also unaware of how much they influence how I raise them, how they impact my worldview, and how they show me how to give love by sharing their love with me. I am a privileged man to have these children in my life who provide for me a living example of how to be a better human being.

At this point in my life I fully realize that fathering, and more importantly Black fathering, biracial children is and encompasses a way of being and navigating a world that does not want or respect who I am as a person. It, in turn, leads me to believe that as a result, my children will be unseen and unheard as they navigate their lives. While on one hand I hold a generalized sense of fear that many parents share, I simultaneously feel an overwhelming burden to prepare my children to be objectified, called exotic as if they were a rug or an item for purchase, or seen as a threat by others who fear them as an unknown. Being biracial, yet seen as Black in times of despair by others, exacerbates my children being unseen and unheard leading to fear of the unknown which is what people greatly fear. In my reality, my children are the poster examples of strong, graceful, resilient, fearless, and powerful, and most days they use their agency in an unapologetic manner.

My greatest hope as their father is that they will always do this. My greatest fear is that the world will wear them down and they will feel powerless to combat it and be without a homeplace to recoup.

As I understand it from bell hooks and other scholars, homeplace is that place on earth where as a human entrenched in the world you can go to this place for respite, rest, gain strength, and foster resilience. More about this will come later.

WHAT DOES FATHERING LOOK LIKE?

At this point in my life, my Black fathering revolves around the notion of preparing my children for a world that does not see them as fitting within a specific label. I feel that it scares people in the world when they are unable to place a label to a person. My children are those persons for whom a label does not squarely fit. My fathering involves raising children who transcend labels and to empower them to embrace the most salient parts of their being and to then try as best they can to shrug off the nonsense of the world. It involves preparing my children to call out and fight the concerns and issues of people who can be small minded, caring, kind, racist, uninformed, ambivalent, ignorant, loving, and confused all at the same time.

My children's needs are simple and complex at the same time. As biracial children I hold the value that they should be raised to embrace all sides of their experiences, identities, and intersectionality. My fear as the father of biracial children is that the rest of the world does not care about their multiple identities and will then marginalize them so that they can label them.

Black fathering to me is to be the provider of preparatory training for my children to embrace being biracial in this world that sees them as Black. Black fathering is preparing my children to be objectified, vilified, and questioned at every turn by others who don't believe in their intellect and intelligence. In addition, my Black fathering is centered on the needs of my children first, then focusing on the outside world. My Black fathering is most importantly grounded in the idea that I must help my children know love by seeing and experiencing it in real life and real time. They have to see and experience the love of their family, the love of their parents, and the love of others. To see it and live with it hopefully provides an experience that they can then live out in their own life in their own way. If I can in some way help them love and respect themselves more than anything else, they are then prepared to combat the challenges of the 21st century and beyond. If I can help them develop creative ways to access their agency, make good decisions, and choose good friends, then I will have helped them develop what bell hooks writes about as homeplace. In my understanding of the construct and stated earlier, homeplace serves as a place of rest and resistance to stimulate resilience. I hope that my children have and continue to find that for themselves whether it be in a church, a barbershop, at home, or with friends. I want them to feel love. I hope that they have people and places in their life that help them energize and feel like they can tackle life's greatest challenges. Black fathering to me in this day looks the same as it did 35 years ago. Black fathering requires me to show up, be present, be emotionally available, nurturing, caring, loving, and preparatory. Black fathering requires consistent love and patience as I guide my children while they in turn guide me to be a better man.

Counseling and support

In this day and time, this question to me is silly, scary, needed, and traumatizing. The question is silly to me because there is no way that each of us could not at one time use even brief counseling to navigate any one of life's many speed bumps. For many of us in the world, our truth is that we don't know enough about it to trust the process. As a Black father I could also see why my children would balk at the prospect of counseling. I can see why Black men balk at the notion of telling their fears, troubles, wants, needs, and desires to a white person who personifies the example of people who don't like Black people. The proposition of counseling is scary because of what has been previously said coupled with the way that Black people seek counsel and support in other healthy ways. At the same time, some people seek support and counsel in unhealthy ways. Finally, the overall question is needed.

My role as a father to biracial children whose mothers are white and Puerto Rican at times brings a stress and that only the parents of biracial children can see because it lives in our home. I have heard people call my daughters exotic as if they were an item for purchase. I have daughters who at an early age had to confront sexism, bullying, and unwanted touches from others before the age of 10. All of these add to the reasons why as a Black father of biracial children, counseling and support would be helpful. My needs can be supported through listening ears from a counselor who will allow me to be myself and serve as an allied accomplice in my journey to maintain health and well-being. My needs are to have an advocate and someone who will say "hell yeah" in their effort to support my experience of being a Black father who is fearful for his own existence in a world that does not love Black men. I then have the same fears for my daughters who are women viewed as objects in this world and subservient to men.

I have in advance cried for my daughters' future experiences of being objectified. I have in advance cried for my son and his future experiences versus his destiny of being a Black boy in America who is literally and figuratively dying to become a Black man in America.

The irony in this is that America has in many ways shown him that they are not fond of him. In some ways whenever a Black boy dies in this country by violence, my son loses a little of his spirit. The Black boy who has died now has no chance to meet my son in high school, in college, or on the subway and transform his life. My son loses in this scenario. He misses out on a significant and meaningful relationship. These are existential and daily issues that a counselor could help me as a growth seeking Black man to explore. Examples like this could serve to positively impact my fathering if my counselor views my perspective as valid. A counselor who challenges and fosters vulnerability would be helpful to the point that they are then able to see and hear the experience of the client as a human who is facing adverse trauma on a daily basis.

What I have learned in my journey through counseling is that my needs are valid. I have learned that it's okay to release the unrealistic expectations of others that hurt my soul, and that my Black life matters. I have learned that as much as my children need to see success in life, they must also learn humility through seeing their father show humility. I learned from my father the power of showing humility and asking forgiveness in the face of a mistake. My father who is also influential in my current fathering apologized daily—once he achieved sobriety—for his actions and inactions as a father to me and husband to my mother. He repeatedly would humbly ask for forgiveness and in his request would with humility state why he was asking for forgiveness. One day when I was in my 20s he asked me if he was a good father. My response to him was simple and to the point. When you were sober, you were the best father on earth. I hope that someday my children will say to me, "You are the best father on earth." My counselor should support me in this journey and challenge me to be the father who I am destined to become. In turn, I have learned that as a father of biracial children and as a Black man in this world, I have needs that I must clearly understand and then express in a way that others can hear me. I know that at times I say "in a way that others can hear me through their fear of me."

WHAT COUNSELORS SHOULD KNOW

Professional counselors should know that their roles are diverse and multifaceted. They have a lot to learn if they are going to be helpful to me. They must learn to always remember that I am a Black man in this world and that my status as a Black man holds value and meaning. My life matters and that I exist to live life in a beautiful and meaningful way. They have to learn the value and meaning of family to me. They have to learn that they will never be me, yet can be helpful to me. They have to learn that they must earn my trust and that their privilege only exists outside of our therapeutic relationship. They do not have the ability to read a chapter in a text about counseling Black men and know who I am, what I stand for, and what I love. As they have read the previous set of words I now want them to check in with themselves and every instance where they said to themselves, "That sounds like something I would do with anyone." I would then want them to ask themselves—was I thinking about how I would do that with a Black father who is raising biracial children? They need to do that.

They need to do that right now.

This is who I am and this is what I do. I am a heterosexual, cisgender, Black man who is raising biracial children in a world where Black people are viewed as being less capable, qualified, or intelligent. I do not believe any of this to be true, yet I live in a world with my children where this thought process exists and is evidenced in some of the most explicit and implicit ways. As professional counselors who will serve Black men who raise biracial children, I feel that it is imperative they begin—in their best way—to understand this and then take action to disrupt this way of thinking and being in the world. Yes, I am calling for them as white counselors to advocate for the human dignity and needs alongside of clients who are Black. I want them to fully realize that the developmental need of Black men raising biracial children in this world differ from those of Black men raising Black children yet at times can be the same. It is their role and responsibility to then gain an understanding of context and nuance. It is their role to be just, humane, and intellectually and clinically curious. This should be balanced with empathy, humanity, humility, and willingness to listen as a means of learning how you can best be helpful to Black men who raising biracial children in the 21st century.

CHAPTER SIX

Fathering Children with Developmental Differences

ERIC WILLIAMS, PHD, LMFT

FATHER PROFILE

Eric Williams has been married to his one true love, Dana since 2006. They have 12-year-old twin boys Carter and Caden both of whom have autism. They also have a three-year-old neurotypical daughter, Erica, who plays big sister and second momma for the twins. Eric is a military veteran and licensed clinical mental health counselor and licensed marriage and family therapist serving service members and their families in the Fayetteville/Ft. Bragg and Raleigh areas of North Carolina. He also serves on the board of directors for both the Autism Society of Cumberland County and Mariposa School for Children with Autism. He blogs about autism and relationship dynamics within couples in his spare time and is an adjunct faculty member at both Touro University Worldwide and Huntington University.

THE GREATEST INFLUENCE ON MY FATHERING

As the oldest of three sons, I was thrust into responsibility for others at a young age. I was responsible for ensuring my brothers didn't go outside when my parents were still at work and responsible for making sure they were awake and ready for school every morning. I was raised in a two-parent home until the age of 13 where

I was exposed to excess alcoholism, verbal abuse, and domestic violence via my father.

I recall telling my mother I "hated" my father numerous times out of pain and frustration.

Needless to say, I did not have the most positive example of what it meant to be a man, let alone a father. Like many families challenged with addiction, apologies were rarely offered. Forgiveness came in the form of keeping everything buried inside with what seemed like a commitment to not ever talking about it.

I learned a lot about who I did not want to become as a father throughout my childhood and that partially shaped the father I am now.

In fact, I grew up wanting to be better than my dad in everything he had ever done even if it was in something he did great. I grew up with a "don't be like dad, be better than dad" mentality without ever having any idea of what healthy fathering really looked like. It would be inaccurate to say my relationship with my dad was strained my entire life; however, the situations from early childhood and adolescence have lingered making it difficult for me to make parenting decisions that resemble decisions or actions he would have taken.

BEFORE FATHERHOOD

"Do you know what those two circles are?" the physician asked my wife and me as we were attending an appointment for our first ultrasound. This was back in 2007, and I was ecstatic and proudly professed to family and friends that we were expecting twins. Bringing a child into the world was a proud moment for me, but learning that I was bringing twin boys into the world made me puff my chest out a little more. For some strange reason, it made me feel a bit more macho.

Growing up as a child who played multiple sports, pledged Phi Beta Sigma Fraternity Inc., and became a paratrooper in the United States Armygave me big dreams for my boys.

I felt an intense sense of purpose and was committed to raising the bar high for them to meet and exceed.

The military taught me that leaders lead by example; therefore, I was committed to living my life as an example (i.e., academic achievement, no police record, financial discipline, etc.) of what they should strive to achieve and surpass. Furthermore, being a Black man in America came with a duffle bag full of negative stereotypes that included being a "baby daddy" versus a husband and father; having multiple children with multiple women; being uneducated; being a drug dealer; dying early, etc. However, one that was most salient was the stereotype of absent Black fathers. I was compelled to further break the stereotype of Black fathers being absent from their kids' lives.

I was raised in a home exposed to alcoholism, domestic violence, and lived through multiple divorces between both parents. I saw a lot of things I didn't want to repeat as a husband and dad. But I also benefitted from positive experiences that I wanted to pass on to my boys. I admit I did not feel the best equipped to be a father to my twins. And what further complicated things was that my road map to fatherhood was filled with instructions about what not to do more than what I thought I should be doing.

THE EARLY YEARS

Twin boys are a handful no matter who you are and what kind of resources you have. Imagine the financial aspect to this. You need double everything: double stroller, two car seats or double sized vehicle, double daycare, double cribs, etc. That macho feeling I once had was short-lived. When I had a moment to breathe, I often asked myself, how will I be able to afford all this and have a life? I remember having a bunch of questions and unfortunately very few answers.

The boys were actually born at 32 weeks as identical twins and spent about a week in the neonatal intensive care unit. It was an indescribable time. Eventually we were sent home with strict orders to feed them every four hours (including throughout the night); it felt like a job but we did it. And we did it with no reservation. As a proud, new father, I did whatever was necessary. Of course, I had the help of my wife, my family, and my stock of Red Bull energy drinks. And I jumped right in and have been there from day one being as versatile as possible.

I have always known the boys' teachers, pediatricians, and have attended appointments. I took them to daycare, made formula, fed them, bathed them, read them stories, etc. You name it, I've done it—a lot. In fact, I have several books etched in my memory right now from reading ro them so often. One consequence of being so involved from the beginning was that I began to notice things about their behaviors and interactions with the world.

Carter, the older of the two by 12 minutes, would scream and cry a lot during the night. We're talking almost colicky, but there was something really troubling him. And this would often result in him awakening Caden as well. This meant both mom and dad were awakened and having poor sleep most nights.

I spent many sleepless nights and early mornings rocking him to sleep while singing nursery rhymes as if I were his "playlist" set to loop over and over.

Eventually, we learned he and Caden both were having constant ear infections. Tubes were eventually implanted in their ears, which seemed to help with their sleep to some extent. However, we later learned this would not be the last experience with the night time awakenings and meltdowns.

Over time, we noticed Carter and Caden would never interact with each other nor with peers at daycare. They appeared to be more isolated and into their very own preferences. Naturally, this put the pressure on me to interact with them individually so that they could have more language and play time. But their language was developing very slowly and so was walking. I began to notice milestones being very delayed, and their preschool teachers when they were as young as two years old began expressing their concerns about their development as well.

"They're fine," I told myself. "I'm going to be patient," I told myself. I shouldn't be concerned because they were born eight weeks premature which was contributing to their hearing problems. That's what I thought. That's what I wanted to believe about why they are delayed. I convinced myself it would be a matter of time.

Then I began to notice the repetitive behaviors (i.e., hand flapping, walking on toes, rocking back and forth, etc.). I noticed the nonverbal noises (i.e., humming, screaming, whining, etc.) they made. And instead of using small sentences to describe what they wanted, they'd just point or use one word like "eat" or "milk."

Here was the issue. As a mental health professional, I knew something was not right. But as a dad, I thought I just have to work harder with them. As a mental health professional, I knew I should seek outside help and guidance from another professional.

As a dad, my pride convinced me there was no way someone else can tell me how to be a good dad.

I knew the system just wanted to label little Black kids anyway and I wasn't having that at all.

In response to this thinking, I literally used to have educational sessions while bathing the boys at night teaching colors, numbers, letters, and reading stories. I'm so serious. I called it the "Daddy's Bathtub Institute." I was determined to work through whatever limitations they were experiencing.

As a Black father raising Black boys in a society where we are stereotyped as being womanizers, violent, baby daddies, and uneducated, it was important for me to disprove those myths and raise my boys to become exceptional men. It was and still is my obligation to ensure they are raised to represent the best image of who God has created them to become and be the men that succeed and inspire others to succeed as well.

MAKING SENSE OF THE DIAGNOSIS

Prior to Carter and Caden's diagnosis, I had heard of autism in a class but nothing significant. The movie Rain Man had come out in 1988 which was 20 years prior to them being born, and I had never watched the movie until years after their diagnosis. In other words, not even Hollywood was able to provide me a slight, or the usual exaggerated and grossly inaccurate, sense of what autism was at that time.

Researchers indicated that autism is an early childhood condition affecting 1 in every 88 children, at that time, where symptoms include deficits in "social-emotional reciprocity," "nonverbal communicative behaviors used for social interaction," and "developing, maintaining, and understand relationships." These symptoms are best considered to be impairments which can seriously limit their successful and age-appropriate functioning in social, occupational, academic, or any other setting they may be expected to successfully navigate. For some individuals with the diagnosis, they may have repetitive patterns of behavior or interests.

My reality was 2:2 children my wife and I procreated had been diagnosed with autism. My wife and I averaged roughly 2–3 hours of continuous sleep before awakening to one or both of them being awake.

Marriage became more of a roommate situation where we loved each other but didn't know how to love each other in the midst of autism.

The thoughts of "people are going to stare" and "Who will care for them if my wife and I die before them?" were and still are present at times. And my ideas about what type of boys and men I'd hoped they'd become had been shattered. Unfortunately, no one I knew was available nor experienced enough to guide me through fathering children with autism nor how to be a husband to a mother of kids with autism. And although they are twins, the diagnosis looked very different between the two of them which meant I was learning how to literally think, read, and speak in two different types of autism.

In addition to the sleepless nights we endured, there was a diminished social life, increased anxiety due to the challenges of leaving my wife alone with two very active and cognitively different children, and the ongoing guilt of whether my wife or I had passed on this diagnosis. New research continued to emerge with the speculation of herbicides, cleaning supplies, age of parents, and vaccinations, to name a few. And while all the speculation about the origins may have been good for some people to know, it was received by me as more reasons how I failed my boys.

Carter and Caden were diagnosed with autism at separate times. Additional diagnoses included: pica, ADHD, seizures, asthma for Caden, and sensory processing disorder. Carter's symptoms were more pronounced than Caden's earning him the diagnosis at roughly two and a half years old. Caden was diagnosed closer to three. That led me to have hope, initially, that only one of them had the diagnosis. But, it turned out we were blessed with two kids with autism.

Having a diagnosis helped us, in my opinion. I remember telling my wife, "I don't care if they call it the 'purple man on the moon syndrome,' at least now we know what we're working with." And I was confident we could get through this. However, at times I blamed myself for my children's diagnosis. Several questions swirled in my mind:

1. "Since I already have a first cousin with severe autism who is institutionalized, is this something I passed on?"
2. "Is this linked to all the shots I had in the military (i.e., small pox, anthrax, yellow fever, etc.)?"
3. "Is my wife going to blame me for their diagnosis?"
4. "How the hell do I parent them?"

My wife had a harder time with the diagnosis. And this only fueled my self-blame and insecurities as a dad. Researchers have suggested mothers of children on the autism spectrum experience much higher emotional and marital distress than fathers (Gau et al., 2012). And the more limited the children's communication skills, the more likely moms experience distress (Baker-Ericzen et al., 2005). This is exactly what was going on in my household since my children were both grossly limited in verbal communication skills. You've likely heard the saying "happy wife, happy life." Well, my wife was emotionally distressed which meant my marriage and happiness followed suit. Needless to say, I began to experience the distress of autism both directly and indirectly. And with there being no cure for autism, I began to question the future quality of life for everyone in my family.

HOW HAS THE DIAGNOSIS INFLUENCED MY MARRIAGE AND FATHERING?

By the time the boys were diagnosed with autism, we'd only been married four years. I was a newly licensed mental health therapist, working full-time in community mental health and starting a private practice. My wife was a top salesperson—a pharmaceutical representative for a Fortune 500 company consistently winning accolades. We were—and are—very driven people.

Autism was very new to us. For first-time parents, parenting—and fathering—can be difficult no matter the circumstances. Parenting twins can be a bit more of a challenge. In my situation, being a first-time father of twins born prematurely who required additional care and later discovering they have a host of developmental diagnoses including autism was mind blowing and relationship rattling. It was as if my wife and I were being thrown every obstacle imaginable.

Being career-driven individuals and having children who attended speech-language therapy (SLT), occupational therapy (OT), and applied behavioral analysis (ABA) therapy, we were stretched thin with very few social supports available. We bore the brunt of the appointments frequently feeling like co-parents or roommates instead of like husband and wife. Feelings of fatigue, isolation, sadness, and overwhelmingness were consistent and strained us severely leaving us unsure how we would do this parenting thing.

And I would be lying if I didn't have the same concerns about how I do this fathering thing.

Now you need to know that insurance didn't cover the Applied Behavioral Analysis (ABA) in school therapy at the time. Nor was the agency we trusted practicing in our city. We commuted one hour each way daily, just to get them to school in a program that charged nearly $2500 per month, per child for half day services. Yes, you read that right! Essentially, the marriage was emotionally, physically, and financially strained in the beginning. Thankfully, counseling and church were very effective in helping us cope.

Over time we became acclimated to life with autism. We learned to make adjustments and necessary sacrifices. We've become advocates for members of the autism community and share the belief that autism is not what happened to us; it's what has inspired us. We both attend the boys' appointments and do our best to support the boys' needs. We share responsibilities of advocating for them and support each other in individual endeavors and time away from the kids. We recognize we need each other for the betterment of our purpose and calling as a couple as well as for the overall greater quality of life for the boys. As a man, I feel a better sense of what it means to be both a husband and father. Here is what I know: my marriage has improved as a result of the improved awareness of autism and how it requires us both to work together.

HAVING A SOCIAL LIFE HELPS ME BE A BETTER FATHER

Can I be honest? I enjoy spending time with my kids as much as I enjoy spending time away from them. The early years were very tough. I didn't feel comfortable leaving my wife with the boys alone due to the challenging nature of the circumstances. And neither of us felt very comfortable trusting other family and friends with the boys. We did not have a long list of family and friends available to assist us; however, my mother-in-law (aka angel-in-law) was readily available.

This short list of people we could trust made it difficult for my wife and I to enjoy friends, family, and each other. Consequently, I began experiencing a significant loss of my identity.

My solution for having a social life was hanging with friends once per week, preferably on a Friday or Saturday night after the kids' bed time. This would also be the time my wife went to bed. Truthfully, I was exhausted, too. But I knew I needed the time with friends even if it only consisted of going to a buddy's house and watching TV. On the way out, I'd drink something caffeinated just to make sure I had enough energy to socialize and make it back home by midnight. Occasionally, I'd go visit my brothers for a weekend, but that'd be no more than twice a year. Doing this helped me to strengthen connections with people I previously enjoyed and regain a sense of the man I once was.

Within the past several years, I've learned to trust more people with the boys; however, it is still a process for me. The boys have innovation waiver services funded by Medicaid, which are, in a nutshell, individuals that have some level of training that provide skill-building services at home and in the community. This, in part, means I have people who I don't know very well come into my home and provide services to my boys daily. This does allow more time to date my wife and occasionally go to professional conferences with colleagues. I also find the time to visit my brothers occasionally and entertain friends and family when they visit.

It can often be awkward when new people ask if I have children. That usually opens up a line of questions pertaining to what school the boys attend or guessing what grade level they are. Explaining this is not an inconvenience, but my response includes an explanation about autism usually resulting in some form of awkwardness on their end. And then there are those unspoken moments of discomfort when I see my peers or family members with whom I am close share pictures or stories on social media with their children who are playing sports, graduating from high school or college, or working their first jobs. I am always happy to see others succeed; however, it also comes at the cost of remembering I have to adjust my definition of success for my kids to be very different from what I initially imagined for them.

How did my children's diagnosis influence my ability to work and financially provide?

I once read the lifetime cost of raising a child with autism without intellectual disabilities is $1.4 million and $2.4 million if the child has intellectual disabilities (Buescher, Cidav, Knapp, & Mandell, 2014). Lucky for us, we had two children diagnosed with autism who also had intellectual disability diagnoses. As a new counselor struggling to get a private practice going in a rural town of North Carolina, I felt an intense amount of pressure to work while also experiencing a significant amount of inadequacy as a father and husband. As a guy who wanted to "fix" the problem, I didn't know how I could fix this situation. And this also created an emotional earthquake within the marriage where we found it difficult to be supportive and connected to each other.

Because my wife was battling post-partum depression for some time in addition to caring for twin boys with autism, working for a Fortune 500 company, and bringing home the bulk of the income, it made it difficult for me to have a desire to pursue more in my career because I wanted to be home more to support her and the kids. And a part of me blamed myself for the boys' diagnosis, my wife's post-partum, and the lack of sufficient income.

Contrary to what might be perceived based on that million-dollar figure above, it's not uncommon for one parent to sacrifice their career within the autism community. The number of medical and mental health appointments per week can be overwhelming for any parent and their employer. I considered not working and taking care of the family so that my wife could pursue her passion in corporate America. Essentially, I was saying "yes" to her dreams and "no" to mine, and that's the tricky part about being a family with autism. But that decision would have only been beneficial for the kids and my wife, to some extent, because I would have sacrificed my professional identity. There's a good chance I would not have been the best parent and husband for the family. As is evident, there wasn't an easy fix for this situation. To make things work I made strategic sacrifices which included not attending professional conferences unless they were within an hour drive of home nor would I network as much with professional colleagues. In fact, I only partially identified as a therapist and primarily as an autism father, and at times I really struggled with how much longer I was going to work as a therapist.

As a private practice therapist, if I didn't work, I didn't bring any money home for the family. And missing time at work for various reasons (i.e. speech therapy, ABA therapy, occupational therapy, neurologist, pediatrician, etc.) was and still is the name of the game when raising children with autism. I did what I had to do while earning whatever income I could make to support my family. Therefore, presenting at conferences, professional networking, mentor groups, etc., were not appealing to me because they either took me away from family or pulled me away from an opportunity to earn more income to support my family.

For a very long time, I struggled with the balance of being a husband, father, and professional. I could never provide enough emotional and financial support for the family nor for the private practice business I had already begun. It's the one thing that still affects me now when I look back at the work–life imbalance then. While I don't regret any of it, I do wish I would have developed a better work–life balance.

HOW HAS THE DIAGNOSIS INFLUENCED MY IDENTITY?

My sense of self was shaken quite a bit as I was learning to rethink what it means to be a dad and husband. There were moments of frustration with the marriage as well as parenting. In fact, there were moments of frustration with myself as well. I didn't know what to do as a parent, husband, nor as a Black man. My kids didn't know what to expect of a dad, but I knew what I had imagined I wanted to be for them and teach them. I'd always believed if I'd set the bar high for my kids through my own life experiences and accomplishments, it would be a way to underscore the lessons I'd like to teach them. Having no police record, no children born out of wedlock, an education, service to the country, and marriage, I wanted to teach my two, young, Black men how to become mature husbands and fathers. It was becoming evident that those were not the lessons I'd be teaching them.

As a husband, like many men in general, I was still trying to figure that out. But being the husband of a Black woman working in corporate America who has twin boys diagnosed with autism was tough. In other words, I knew she had to be on her A game daily for work. But the challenges of autism were difficult for both of us. And like many decent husbands, I wanted to fix the issues, or in this case the autism, for her. But I couldn't. And that left me feeling helpless, afraid, and alone because I couldn't fix the autism for the twins nor for my wife. And the question I struggled with was "What kind of husband or father am I if I can't meet the needs of my wife and kids?"

As times have progressed, I've learned that I don't need to fix the diagnosis. I only need to fix my thinking.

I have learned to accept the diagnosis for what it is and the impact it has on my family. I still struggle with the moments of helplessness, fear, and being alone, but I also understand that those emotions are part of the process for most special needs parents. Parents of children diagnosed with autism experience much higher levels of emotional distress to include anxiety and depression than parents of neurotypical children (Benson & Karlof, 2009; Bitsika & Sharpley, 2004). Furthermore, parents feel stretched beyond their limits and incapable of coping (Bitsika, Sharpley, & Bell, 2013). I accept that. I accept that who I am, how I meet the needs of my family, and how I interact with the rest of the world is simply unique, and like a tide, my emotions will ebb and flow.

ADVICE FOR BLACK FATHERS OF CHILDREN WITH AUTISM

This is usually a tough question to answer. In the autism community, one will commonly hear some version of, "When you see one child with autism, you only see one child with autism." In other words, autism doesn't look the same in every child. In fact, my identical twin boys have very different needs and require different parenting strategies. Their symptoms are not identical nor are the medications they take.

I have learned that it's true that not all children with autism are the same and not all families of children with autism are the same either. In other words, to paraphrase the earlier statement, "When you see one family of a child with autism, you only see one family of a child with autism." I didn't know what I needed from others nor how to obtain it. I lacked the social supports to assist me with the emotionally stressful moments of parenting autism, and at times I struggled with symptoms of depression and anxiety.

Looking back, I cried out for help in ways that masked what I was truly feeling and engaged in behaviors that negatively affected my marriage.

I wish I had gone to counseling to sort out some of the emotions I was experiencing prior to acting out in ways that hurt my marriage. And I wish I had known of a social support system of other men that were experiencing life as an autism dad. My pride, the desire to fix autism instead of working on myself, and the idea that earning more money was more important than spending it on a counselor kept me from becoming being the family man I needed to be. I would not advise any man to repeat what I've done.

When I think about advice I'd offer a new Black fathers who has discovered he has a child with autism, my first advice would be to seek the counsel of others. This could be professional counselors, pastors, parenting experts, etc. Get the necessary help for yourself and your family and don't suffer in silence. You can't do this alone, and you don't have to. Remember, real men go to counseling. And counseling saves lives and relationships including those affected by autism.

Another piece of advice I'd suggest is focusing on what your child as well as their partner needs instead of comparing your child and family to that of others. Simply put, your child and family are not less than, just differently-abled than some others. And because they are differently abled, they require different needs. All they need from you is to know and experience you as a differently capable man.

My final piece of advice would be to find a quote, philosophy, or scripture that helps you stay grounded through the tough times. This can be anything that keeps you driven to be present in the lives of those around as well as to take better care of yourself to prolong how long you can remain in the lives of your loved ones. In the beginning when I blamed myself for the diagnosis, I found two very powerful Biblical scriptures:

1. Then the Lord said to him, "Who has made man's mouth? Who makes him mute, or deaf, or seeing, or blind? Is it not I, the Lord?"—Exodus 4:11 (ESV)
2. As he passed by, he saw a man blind from birth. And his disciples asked him, "Rabbi, who sinned, this man or his parents, that he was born blind?" Jesus answered, "It was not that this man sinned, or his parents, but that the works of God might be displayed in him."—John 9:1–3 (ESV)

These scriptures allowed me to let go and let God.

As I've continued to let God, I stumbled across a quote that has helped reshape my thinking about my family and myself both personally and professionally:

> The life I touch for good or ill will touch another life, and in turn another, until who knows where the trembling stops or in what far place my touch will be felt.
>
> —Frederick Buechner

As a Black father, your existence means so much to so many people whether you know them directly or indirectly. You are touching lives every moment of everyday. The influence you have on your family will be felt by others with whom they come into contact. And this ripple effect will continue outward onto other people you may never meet. Will your ripple effect be something positive or negative? Find the encouraging thoughts or words that inspire you to be present even during the toughest of times so that your influence on their lives can be felt far beyond your imagination.

REFERENCES

Baker-Ericzen, M. J., Brookman-Frazee, L., & Stahmer, A. (2005). Stress levels and adaptability in parents of toddlers with and without autism spectrum disorders. *Research and Practice for Persons with Severe Disabilities*, *30*, 194–204. doi:10.2511/rpsd.30.4.194

Benson, P. R., & Karlof, K. L. (2009). Anger, stress proliferation, and depressed mood among parents of children with ASD. A longitudinal replication. *Journal of Autism and Developmental Disorders*, *39*, 350–362.

Bitsika, V., & Sharpley, C. F. (2004). Stress, anxiety and depression among parents of children with autism spectrum disorder. *Australian Journal of Guidance and Counselling*, *14*, 151–161.

Bitsika, V., Sharpley, C., & Bell, R. (2013). The buffering effect of resilience upon stress, anxiety and depression in parents of a child with an autism spectrum disorder. *Journal of Developmental & Physical Disabilities*, *25*(5), 533–543. doi:10.1007/s10882-013-9333-5

Buescher, A.V. S., Cidav, Z., Knapp, M., & Mandell, D. S. (2014). Costs of autism spectrum disorders in the United Kingdom and the United States. *JAMA Pediatrics*, *168*(8), 721–728. https://doi.org/10.1001/jamapediatrics.2014.210

Gau, S. S., Chou, M., Chiang, H., Lee, J., Wong, C., Chou, W., & Wu, Y. (2012). Parental adjustment, marital relationship, and family function in families of children with autism. *Research in Autism Spectrum Disorders*, 6263–270. doi:10.1016/j.rasd.2011.05.007

CHAPTER SEVEN

Renegotiating Relationships with Emerging Adolescents

REV. ROBERT C. ROGERS, MA, LAC, NCC

FATHER PROFILE

Robert Rogers is a licensed associate counselor (NJ) and a national certified counselor. He serves as a pastor and professional counselor working to empower people of color to combat systemic racism and internalized oppression and equip both congregants and clients to overcome obstacles to growth, fulfill their potential, and live authentic and meaningful lives. He is currently a doctoral candidate in counseling with a concentration in spirituality and counseling. He has served as a hospital chaplain, hospice chaplain, and bereavement group facilitator. He has served in his present pastoral position at a Pentecostal church for 25 years. Robert is divorced and the proud father of Khiana, 22, and Kendall, 20, both of whom are college students.

BIGGEST INFLUENCES ON MY FATHERING

My father, Gordon Anthony Rogers, existed as the biggest influence on my fathering as evidenced by the fatherhood I have practiced. Born in 1919 in a small, suburban New Jersey town as the first born of eight children, my father was part of the "greatest generation," those men and women born between 1910 and 1928, who grew up during the Great Depression and served in World War

II. Tom Brokaw (2014), NBC News anchor and commentator who created the phrase greatest generation described these men and women as "the greatest generation any society ever produced: [they] survived the Depression, won the War, came home and built the country we have today." Returning home from the war, my father worked for 45 years at Lobel's Youth Center, a children's clothing store, as a stock manager, but in actuality as the store manager. He further served as an assistant pastor in the Church of God in Christ for over 20 years and then served as pastor for 30 years until his death in 1995.

While not many detailed accounts are known about his growing up, by his own accounts he experienced some bullying in school and grew up in poverty. What distinguished him from other students and siblings was his analytical, mechanical mind and acute grasp of math and accounting whereby he won the Accounting Award in high school. His mechanical abilities enabled to him to repair machinery, equipment, or cars. Inducted into the army in 1945, he served in the 580th Ordnance Ammunition Company in World War II in the Philippines. His mechanical and analytical abilities led him to be put in charge of their unit's supplies—accounting for, managing, and dispatching them. What is further significant about his analytical abilities is that these abilities have been passed down to his children, which have allowed us to be successful academically and professionally. I have incorporated these abilities into how I approach the world of relationships, including my fathering, by focusing primarily on thoughts and tasks rather than feelings.

My father was a stickler for rules, being on time, and getting work done. Following the rules and respecting authority were an integral part of his personality. He probably learned this from his own father, Luther, and living in large family of eight children which at times included additional foster children. This translated into our family with my siblings and me doing what we each were assigned to do, especially getting our household chores and homework done before engaging in any leisure time. In our home he coined the phrase, "Stay in your own lane," which meant each person doing what they were supposed to do without infringing on another person's responsibilities or telling that person what they ought to be doing. However, the focus on work was not only on getting things done but also done in the right way and completely; things could not be "half done" as he would say. Another way he conveyed the importance of taking initiative and being responsible was by telling us, "Your tail will be glad when your body is dead for forever sitting on it."

Naturally, this emphasis on getting work done, done right, and well the first time was socialized into us as children. My siblings and I would quote the following saying to each other: "If a task is once begun, never leave it until it's done. Be the labor, great or small, do it well or not at all." As a result, I learned the work ethic of completing tasks, doing them thoroughly and well, fulfilling my responsibilities without being told what and how to do, and making sure work was done before enjoying leisure time activities. All of these values influenced my fathering. I focused on getting things done in the house making sure the children were taken care of and the children were doing what they were supposed to be doing, such as getting homework done.

My father always wanted to be on time and never late; punctuality was a sign of virtue, responsibility, excellence, and character and what it really meant was always being early. He would be on time—or early—to open up the children's clothing store and set things in order and ensure the cleanliness of the sidewalk and entrance. This also translated into his pastoral leadership. It was common practice for him, my mother, and us children to go to a weeknight church service and arrive ten minutes early. My father would start singing and my mother would start playing the piano when the clock struck 7:30 pm, even if no other members were present. Then he would start praying and members would eventually arrive.

Even though he never admitted it to me, I believe that he wanted to defy the stereotype that Black people are always late. He never embraced the idea of "CP time" or colored peoples' time. In whatever area of life of being somewhere, it was a must to be on time. This penchant for being on time has rubbed off on me, too. I, too, will arrive early for meetings, appointments, and classes. Deep down inside I like being on time and disproving the existence of "CP time." I have raised my children with this same value of being on time.

My father provided both a moral compass and spiritual foundation for us being in the world. Undergirded by his faith in and personal relationship with God, my father demonstrated a highly moral Christian lifestyle based upon the precepts of the Bible and tenets of Pentecostal-Holiness doctrine. For him (and our mother) this translated into a lifestyle of no drinking, smoking, dancing, cursing, listening to secular music, partying, or going to movies. Our parents' priority was living a life pleasing to God and having a positive influence on the world through their Christian lifestyle, which provided us children with a moral and spiritual foundation upon which to function in the world.

We, too, embraced and practiced a Christian lifestyle in our childhood and adolescent years, which in truth was instilled within us with limited engagement with the broader, cultural world. Our lives consisted primarily of home, church, school, and sports with little time for much else. Of course, upon leaving home and entering our college years gave us more exposure to the world and opportunity to choose our own values and lifestyle. What we made of our lives was based on our choices and responsibility to be the author of our lives. However, in order to build our lives successfully, we needed a solid foundation of morals, values, and healthy behaviors, which our father provided. As a father raising my own children, I have often reflected on these questions: What are my core values or principles that are non-negotiable and guide my daily interactions? What are my ethical principles or standards, which provide a moral compass and grounding for the choices I make? How do I live out these values and principles in my world of relationships and especially in front of my children?

This moral and spiritual foundation has shaped my fathering in that I have tried to provide core values, moral and ethical principles, and a spiritual example and foundation to my children. Examples of core values included accepting and respecting people regardless of their race/ethnicity and cultural background and respecting/honoring elders.

Moral and ethical principles can be summed up in doing the right thing for the right reason at the right time and hopefully with the right motivation.

Even if my children may not have had the right motivation, I encouraged them to do the right thing anyway. These principles further included making good choices, which lead to positive consequences, and being a leader and not a follower by not allowing others to blindly lead or influence them. The spiritual foundation provided to my children included exposure to my Christian faith and its practices. For example, I taught my children the Lord's Prayer when they were toddlers. In fact, when I drove them to daycare each morning, I would say the Lord's Prayer with them not only for them to learn the Lord's Prayer but also learn the value of prayer as a spiritual resource to start one's day. I further taught them to say prayers at bedtime and before meals. My children attended church services and participated in children's programs, such as Sunday School and children's choir.

Dedication was the singular characteristic that epitomized my father—dedication to family, God, country, church, and work. When examining his life, this trait and theme of dedication and faithfulness runs clearly throughout his life. In our counseling profession this value is described as fidelity, that is, "honoring commitments and keeping promises, including fulfilling one's responsibilities of trust" (American Counseling Association, 2014, p. 3). Moreover, my father's dedication included the element of sacrifice, giving of oneself, especially one's time and resources, for the well-being of others. For my father this spirit of dedication included helping people, organizations, and anyone who asked him for a helping hand, especially money.

While he gave and loaned people several thousands of dollars, needless to say, he very rarely received repayment of those loans. One lesson I definitely learned from this was to not get into providing loans to people!

However, his example of dedication to his family influenced me in making sure I demonstrated the same level of dedication and support to my children. My father financially supported his mother and sister, Nadine, who lived in Lakewood, New Jersey, and often visited them. When needed and requested, he would support his other brothers. Regarding his own immediate family, my father supported us to the highest degree and made sacrifices of which we were not always aware. As a result, we were lacking very little throughout our childhood, adolescence, and young adulthood. His support and sacrifice even continued into our adulthood. His dedication and sacrifice influenced me significantly by providing me with a clear example of fathering to provide for and support my children.

As part of the greatest generation and growing up in his family of origin, my father developed a solid work ethic and contributed to stabilizing and improving his world of family, work, and church. He personified a personality of a strong, quiet type, who fulfilled his responsibilities of working hard and providing for our family. He was a consistent presence and pillar for our family, which included dinnertime meals and him leading us in prayer before leaving the house each morning. However, my father had little, personal interaction, conversation, and emotional engagement with us children, especially with me as the youngest child. Moreover, with him working at the children's clothing store during the daytime and working in church ministry after work, he had no time to attend any of our sports or extracurricular activities. It was our mother who drove us to and attended these activities. This influenced my fathering in that I was determined to attend and participate in my children's activities in their childhood and adolescent years.

This meant that I had to set boundaries and limits in my work life as a pastor, which my father did not do, so that I could be available to spend time with the children at home and participate in their school, sports, and extracurricular activities. In addition, I wanted to be able to communicate and connect with my children on a personal level.

In May 1987 after graduating from Columbia University Business School, I returned home to accept a job in corporate finance with AT&T. However, it was not the happenstance of a job search, as I first thought, which brought me back to my hometown and home church, but God's providence brought me back to assist my father in ministry and develop a personal relationship with him. In the eight years before he died, I worked with my father in our church taking on administrative and planning responsibilities to lighten his workload as he continued to age and decline in health. This included driving him to denominational meetings in Trenton, New Jersey, several times during the year. This working relationship provided the opportunity to develop a more personal relationship with him, which I did not have in my younger years. On the evening of June 25, 1995, I visited my father for the last time, with him dying at his home, and then returned to my home. After falling asleep, I had a dream of my father driving the church van with me in the passenger seat next to him. Suddenly a bright light came from behind the van with the light shining so brightly that the reflection in the rearview mirror was hurting my father's eyes. I tried to block the light's intensity by putting my hand in front of the mirror but that did not buffer the light's penetrating brightness. Then the telephone rang waking me from sleep and my sister told me my father had died. I was blessed to get to know my father in the last eight years of his life. As I looked forward to my own fatherhood, my hope and prayer were that I would have a personal relationship with my children long before the closing years of my life arrived.

I inherited not only my father's style of dedication, presence, and support but also his introverted personality and its lack of outward, active emotional, interpersonal engagement that my children needed, which became my growing edge, challenge, and priority to work on. Kottler (2010) described the irony of being a counselor in how we treat clients compared to sometimes how we may treat our own family members. For example, as counselors we give our clients full, undivided attention which we may not give consistently to our family members. Kottler's reflection seemed parallel to the public folklore tale of the shoemaker whose children did not have any shoes. The challenge came for me to provide the attention, active listening, emotional responsiveness, and perspective that I thought my children needed. This whole idea of perspective included sharing my unique experiences, lessons I have learned, information, and wisdom to equip them to live effectively without repeating my mistakes if possible.

My goal, and I believe the goal of Black fathering, is to equip our children with sufficient knowledge, wisdom, common sense, awareness, critical thinking skills, self-confidence, and emotional and spiritual support in order for them to thrive in their world.

WHAT DOES BLACK FATHERING LOOK LIKE NOW?

As our children grow up, it is natural for parents to look at and admire them for their growth and development. However, when the emergent adolescents' years arrive, sometimes we may ask the question, "Who are these people"? It is during these years that our children are growing and becoming their own unique selves. Sometimes that unique self clashes with our expectations and vision of who our children are and who we think they are becoming or should become. While they may resemble us in appearance and physical features, their social and emotional development in today's world may surprise us.

Who are these adolescent young people? They are Generation Z! I met the first two of this generation in 1998 and 1999 when my two children were born 18 months apart. Generation Z consists of those young people who were born between 1997 and 2012, which would make them ages 8 to 23 in 2020 (Dimock, 2019). When the 9/11 attack on the World Trade Center occurred in 2001, my children were three and a half and two years old in a daycare center. When

President Barack Obama took office in January 2009, my children were 11 and 9 years old in elementary school. The prior generation before Generation Z is the Millennial Generation, who were born between 1981 and 1996 (Dimock, 2019). The Pew Research Center described Generation Z as more diverse with 48% being nonwhite compared to 39% nonwhite in the Millennial Generation (Fry & Parker, 2018). In further comparison to Millennials, Generation Z had a lower high school drop-out rate and higher college enrollment (Fry & Parker, 2018).

Generation Z members described their lived experiences and acknowledged the major problems they are facing to include anxiety and depression, bullying, drug addiction, drinking alcohol, poverty, teenage pregnancy, and gangs (Geiger & Davis, 2019; Horowitz & Graf, 2019). For those Generation Z members 13–17 in 2018, they further acknowledged "feeling tense or nervous about their day everyday or almost every day" with 36% of girls and 23% of boys reporting this (Horowitz & Graf, 2019, p. 3). The Pew Research Center further found that these youth reported their daily experience included feeling bored (40%), wanting more good friends (29%), being put down by people (24%), concerned about their families having enough money (23%), and being targeted by law enforcement (7%) (Horowitz & Graf, 2019). Thirty-five percent of girls and 23% of boys experienced "a lot of pressure to look good" as well as the pressure to fit in socially and get good grades (Horowitz & Graf, 2019, p. 3).

Erikson (1963, 1968) described the central task of adolescence as establishing a clear sense of one's identity and where one fits in the world. Designating this psychosocial stage as identity versus role confusion, Erikson posited that the unsuccessful achievement of identity will result in role confusion of what the adolescent is to do with their life. Erikson further posited that achieving a solid ego identity prepares adolescents for successful functioning in the adult world of responsibilities and relationships and supports positive mental health outcomes and social adaptation. Marcia (1996) underscored the importance of youth actively exploring, wrestling with, and successfully achieving an identity.

For Black youth, developing such an ego identity remains challenging at best given their present existence in a racist society which daily confronts and invalidates Black identity through racial microaggressions (Bang, 2015; Sue et al., 2008). These same youth face the additional challenge of establishing an ethnic identity of who am I as part of a specific ethnic group and what that ethnic group membership means as they figure out where they fit in the world (St. Louis & Liem, 2005). St. Louis and Liem (2005) reported that "ethnic identity is a salient factor in the psychosocial well-being of ethnic minority youth" (p. 242) and they "must integrate both an ego and ethnic identity to develop a positive self-concept" (p. 241). Research has shown that a positive ethnic identity supports successful social adaptation and provides a buffering factor against racial discrimination (St. Louis & Liem, 2005; Tynes, Umana-Taylor, Rose, Lin, & Anderson, 2012).

Given who these emerging adolescents are and their experiences in the world, how can Black fathers support their growth and development?

Affirming ethnic identity

Black fathers can affirm the ethnic identity of their adolescent children and support them in their process of ego identity formation. When the validity of being Black in America is constantly challenged, invalidated, and negated loudly and clearly, Black fathers must affirm and validate their children's racial and ethnic identities not only to our children but also to the social structures in which our children participate, such as in schools. To our children, we affirm their gifts, talents, abilities, academic, athletic, and extracurricular accomplishments, and what is unique about them as these are displayed in everyday interactions. We affirm that Blackness with all of its shades is beautiful. To social systems, we question and challenge any indirect or direct statements or actions, unintentional or intentional, which may be an assault on our children's race/ethnicity, worth, uniqueness, abilities, and rightful place in that social system. For example, during my children's school years, I questioned teacher comments and administrator's behaviors directed at not only my children but also other children of color.

Black fathers can further support their children in their ethnic identity formation by talking with them about what it means to be Black in America and processing our children's experiences of race and ethnicity. My son had an encounter with a lacrosse teammate when his teammate used the word "nigger." My son confronted the teammate directly and appropriately at the time of the incident by addressing him and his ignorance with why that statement was inappropriate, insulting, and degrading while at the same time exercising emotional restraint and a level head. He and I processed the encounter and how he dealt with it. Expressing some concern about the racial attitudes of some other players, we considered other actions he could take to address the culture of the team. He talked with team captains, who had not addressed the incident. Then he talked with the coach, who did address it with the whole team. We thought about other possible strategies, like getting support from other players of color. I also emphasized to him the importance of not letting anyone derail or distract him from pursuing his dreams and passions like playing college lacrosse.

Another important strategy Black fathers can employ is discussing current events involving and impacting people of color which are reported on the internet and television. The goal here is to help our children understand the world they are living in with an insight into the power dynamics and racist strategies underlying these events. I routinely have sent articles from the New York Times, such as "The Racial Bias Built into Photography" in which Sarah Lewis (2019) examined the racial bias against dark-skinned people when my son was taking a college photography course. I sent an opinion article by Brent Staples (2019), NY Times editorial board member, entitled, "How Blackface Feeds White Supremacy." In my text accompanying the article link, I said to my children, "This article contains some very important Black history with serious implications on what's happening in today's world. It is a must read!" My purpose in sending this and other articles is to prepare you both for the real world, a world filled with opportunities and challenges; a world in which racism is alive and being nurtured by the current White House. Love, Dad." My commitment to them in deepening their understanding of the world was further demonstrated by me even signing my children up to receive the New York Times weekly newsletter of articles on race, Race/Related.

An additional strategy included learning from the experiences of Black people in the news, which contained both positive and negative lessons. On the positive side, I sent articles about Black people making a difference in the world, like Senator Kamala Harris and Senator Cory Booker. These articles further included stories about important Black people who died, such as Congressman Elijah Cummings, author Toni Morrison, and actress Diahann Carroll, and others who were significant contributors to Black history. I hoped that these positive stories of Black achievement and everyday greatness would deepen my children's appreciation of and pride in their Black heritage as well as inspire them to make their own unique contribution in the world. On the negative side, I shared articles and discussed Black persons who made serious errors in judgment and poor choices for which they suffered consequences. These discussions focused both on ordinary, everyday people and famous people with the hope that my children would learn from these persons' mistakes and help them practice thinking through their own decision-making before implementing unwise choices.

Supporting Identity exploration

In supporting my children through their exploration and working to achieve an ego identity, my goal has been that they would become the unique persons God created them to be. I did not want them to become what I wanted them to be (as some parents do) or follow in my career footsteps. For example, my son was active in the church during his high school years. Some congregants were wondering, maybe even hoping, and encouraging him to follow in my footsteps in ministry. However, I made a clear, public statement to the congregation to not even suggest to him that he follow in my footsteps but allow God and Kendall to decide the direction of his life.

My daughter, Khiana, excelled in STEM (science, technology, engineering, math) classes in high school and expressed an interest in engineering, a field in which Black females represented 1% of undergraduate students in engineering programs in 2017. My job has been to encourage and cheer her on in her pursuit of a degree in mechanical engineering. Moreover, in this supportive role I have had conversations with each of them processing questions about career choices, course selections, and work experiences. This role has further included raising questions, providing alternative perspectives, encouraging them to seek additional information, helping them think through their options and choices, and empowering them to make their own choices and decisions.

Lessons on Driving While Black

One of the milestones of adolescence includes obtaining a driver's permit and license. As evidenced especially over the past few years with the deaths of Black men and women drivers by law enforcement, driving can be challenging and life-threatening if you are Black. Such a precarious and anxiety-producing environment creates the real possibility that a Black person may leave home and not return on any given day due to driving while Black. With all the Black people being murdered by police, I told my son one day as we were driving that my job was three-fold: (1) to keep him alive, (2) to keep him out of jail, and (3) to help him graduate from college. As a Black father, all of this means teaching my children the skills necessary to lower the chances of being stopped by police and what to do when stopped. To lower the risks of being stopped by police, I have instructed my children to drive the speed limit, especially on the highway, stay in the right lane except for passing another vehicle, avoid erratic driving patterns, obey the traffic laws, and no distracted driving of any kind.

While these are good driving tips, they still may get stopped just because they are Black. When stopped, I have advised them to have their license and insurance card readily available without having to search or reach for them, keep their hands visible on the steering wheel, no sudden reaching or movements, provide simple, short answers to any questions, and do not agree to any search of the vehicle. While I consider my children responsible drivers, I pray for their safety and protection, especially that they will not have an encounter with the police which will be life threatening. Since driving while Black is such ongoing reality and continuing threat to our children, Black fathers must make this a high priority with our children no matter how long they have been driving nor how old they get.

Offering Wisdom to Navigate the World of Adult Relationships

As Generation Z gets older in their 20s, they may be entering the world of intimate relationships according to Erikson's (1963, 1968) stage of intimacy versus isolation. After forming their identity in the identity versus role confusion stage, persons are now open to connecting and developing more personal, close relationships and even willingly committing to a deeper level of relationship, such as marriage or partnership (Erikson, 1963, 1968).

How do we, Black fathers, talk to our children (or grandchildren) about the world of relationships, especially when it is a subject that is very personal and private to them as well as they may question how much we really know given our place in a different generation? They may further question or doubt our wisdom when, like in my case, having experienced a divorce from their mother. I do not propose easy answers to this question. What may be helpful to this generation is for us to share what we have learned from our own experiences—both good and bad—in relationships as general principles or perspectives to think about. When it has been difficult to share my own experience or when my children may not have wanted to hear my experience, I have resorted to using the experiences of others, persons in the public spotlight or persons they may know. For example, with my son, I have cited the examples of college and professional football players who engaged in dating violence, sexual assault, and intimate partner violence to teach him the importance of respect for women. I have further used and adapted insights from the counseling literature as a lens for them to think about their relationships.

Parrott and Parrott (2015), in their work with dating, engaged, and married couples, proposed a framework to evaluate a couple's relationship at any given point in time by asking each other to rate their relationship on a scale of 1–10 in terms of passion, intimacy, and commitment. Passion represented the physical dimension, intimacy the emotional dimension, and commitment the intellectual dimension (Parrott & Parrott, 2015). While this framework depicted as a triangle may be a helpful tool for some couples to begin having such a conversation to evaluate their relationship, the limitation of this framework is its lack of clarity and delineation of what the scale (1–10) really measures. I have revised their framework by (1) renaming the passion side as physical contact and the intimacy side of the triangle as knowing each other and (2) providing a 1–10 scale for each side of the triangle (see Figure 1) where the higher number indicates an increasing level in that dimension.

The Physical Contact scale depicts increasing levels of physical contact from no physical contact to having sex. The Knowing Each Other scale describes the increasing depth of communication and openness from talking in clichés to communicating on the level of transparency and soul mates. Kelly (2005) proposed seven levels of communication or intimacy, which are the first seven levels on the Knowing Each Other scale, which include clichés, facts, opinions, hopes/dreams, feelings, faults/fears/failures, and legitimate needs. The Commitment Scale describes increasing levels of commitment from basic respect to being in a covenant relationship, such as marriage or partnership.

Physical Contact
1. No touching
2. Shaking Hands
3. Kissing on the cheek
4. Church hug
5. Holding hands
6. Kissing on lips
7. Body hug/embrace
8. French kiss
9. Touching
10. Having sex

Knowing Each Other
1. Clichés
2. Facts
3. Opinions
4. Hopes & dreams
5. Feelings
6. Faults, fears & failures
7. Needs
8. Vulnerabilities
9. Hurts/Pains
10. Transparency/ Soul Mates

Commitment: (1) Respect; (2) Acceptance; (3) Cooperation; (4) Trust; (5) Sharing/Giving; (6) Consistency; (7) Attachment; (8) Dependability/Faithfulness; (9) Sacrifice; (10) Covenant

Figure 1. Understanding Our Relationships

One implication of Figure 1 is that there are a variety of relationships one may have with different combinations of physical contact, knowing each other (communication), and commitment. For example, a relationship with co-workers or colleagues may involve Levels 1–4 on the Physical Contact side, Levels 1–4 in Knowing Each Other, and Levels 1–4 in Commitment. It is important for our children to understand that all relationships are not the same, and each requires clear definition on the part of both participants. A second implication may be that persons can deepen their relationship over time by increasing their levels of knowing each other, commitment, and physical contact, which mean that relationships, which are important to us, require attention and work to grow and develop.

A third implication derives from depicting this model as an equilateral triangle whose equal sides convey the idea of balance. Parrot and Parrot (2015) presented an excellent discussion on balance in relationships using their passion-intimacy-commitment triangle image and the potential results when one of these dimensions predominates over the other two. In addition to this notion of balance, the goal of intimate relationships is also wellness. Hettler (1976) posited social wellness as living in community with others by possessing harmony with them, engaging in healthy communication, and contributing to the welfare of others, the community, and the environment. Building upon Hettler (1976), Roscoe (2009) described wellness in relationships as including (1) quality and skill of interaction, (2) interdependence, (3) giving and receiving support, and (4) self-awareness and other awareness.

With this framework in mind, I have talked with members of both Generation Z and the Millennial Generation, especially those who were dating and contemplating a more serious, committed relationship and those engaged to be married, about their relationships. With a sense of curiosity, I have asked them to define their relationships, the meaning and significance the relationship holds for them, where they think the relationship is going, where they would like it to grow, and how they plan to achieve their desired level of relationship growth and quality. For example, in one case where their relationship included the Touching (9) and Having Sex (10) Levels of Physical Contact, Clichés (1) and Opinions (3) Levels of Knowing Each Other, and the Respect (1) Level of Commitment, I explored with them how they defined and understood their relationship and the relationship's degree of balance or wellness. As interested and concerned fathers, we too can sincerely ask such nonjudgmental questions such as: (1) How is your relationship going?; (2) On what level are you communicating?; (3) How do you see your relationship growing?; (4) What is your level of commitment?: and, (5) How much are they willing to commit to the relationship going forward?

While this framework in Figure 1 lacks empirical validation, it may serve as a tool to stimulate our children's or grandchildren's thinking about the meaning of being in an intimate relationship and encourage conversation with their partners about the nature of their relationships. Such reflection may even open the door for conversations with us fathers to share our wisdom from our own successful, broken, and failed relationships. Even though my children have the freedom and autonomy to choose their own friends and intimate relationships, my hope is that learning from my relationship experiences will provide a little guidance for them to better navigate in their own world of relationships. More importantly, whatever our history of past relationships may have been, hopefully through our present world of relationships, as Black fathers, we can model for our children how healthy relationships are practiced and lived out on a daily basis.

Providing a Hospitable Place in a Hostile World

As a Black father and a counselor, I realize the stressors and challenges my children are facing during these adolescent years and now as they move into young adulthood. As indicated above from the Generation Z data (Desilver, 2019; Geiger & Davis, 2019; Horowitz & Graf, 2019), this generation is facing various pressures and life experiences which are negatively impacting their well-being as evidenced by their own reports of anxiety, depression, and other forms of emotional distress. As a Black father, I try to provide a safe, hospitable space where my children can be present with me in open, honest, and nonjudgmental conversation to talk about their lives. I use the word "hospitable" to describe a space or atmosphere where they are free to be themselves without any demands or pressures to be anyone but themselves. Nouwen (1975) described hospitality as a free and friendly space where people can enter as strangers, interact and connect with others, be themselves, and experience change. Nouwen's description of hospitality seems very fitting in being a father to this generation because at times our children do seem like strangers as we wonder who they are and who they are becoming.

Since the peer group has more influence and power in the lives of adolescents than parents and with them, spending most of their free time with peers, parents and children can seem like strangers at times. However, Black fathers can offer a safe space where our adolescent and young adult children can enter when they choose and receive acceptance, encouragement, affirmation, a listening ear, moral/spiritual strength, perspective, and wisdom. I even try to create this space when I call them to check in. Or, I try to create it even through text messages. Even though we may be miles apart, I remind them that I love them, care what is happening with them, and I am a supportive presence in their lives.

COUNSELING SUPPORT NEEDED/RECEIVED TO NAVIGATE THIS TIME

Five years ago, I re-entered counseling to increase my own personal growth. When I say I re-entered counseling, it means that I had previously sought counseling and then went for additional counseling to address any negative mental, emotional, or relational issues, which prevented me from living an authentic and meaningful life. For example, in 2008 I went into counseling after my divorce from my children's mother in order to heal and adjust to a new life as a single father with parenting responsibilities. That counseling experience helped me to decide to pursue my master's degree in counseling later that year. Then in the end of 2012 when I completed my master's degree, I sought career counseling to review my career in ministry and explore possible options of integrating my counseling training into my work as a pastor. I view life as a life-long journey of growing and learning, becoming one's true self, and realizing your full potential. Just as one takes a car in for a tune-up or one goes to the doctor for a checkup, every now and then I believe that it is important to seek additional insight through counseling to address any blockages to growth or deal with any pressing issues or concerns that might impede my living and working effectively. Therefore, I have sought counseling, not because of any problems with my children, but rather to address issues within myself so that I could be a better person, parent, and pastor.

My purpose in entering counseling was to work more on fulfilling my potential, pursuing my dreams, and living a more effective, authentic, and meaningful life with greater self-awareness and intentionality, especially to make the most of the remaining years of my lifetime. I further sought counseling because I wanted to be more of my true self and be more in touch with how and what I felt, what I thought, valued, wanted, and most of all, be my authentic self in all of my relationships. I did not want people to have to guess what I meant, who I am, what I felt, or what was important to me. But in all of my interactions I wanted consistency and clarity in terms of how I related to people. Since I am more cognitive than emotional, I started to keep a feelings diary throughout the day so that I could more easily identify and be in touch with what I was feeling in the moment. I tried to be more mindful of what was happening inside of me and processing that so that I could respond appropriately, consistently, and conclusively to those feelings as I experienced them. In contrast to my introverted personality, my further goal was also to be more open, direct, proactive, and vulnerable in appropriate ways in my respective relationships. I believed that if I accomplished these goals then this would not only impact my growth but also improve the relationship with my children.

With this agenda and goals in mind, I approached each counseling session proactively by setting the agenda for each session and bringing in specific materials to discuss and work on. These materials included interpersonal interactions, conflict situations, significant conversations, and experiences with the children, dreams, anxieties, and work stressors. The counselor provided an objective sounding board to challenge my thinking and actions and deepen my self-awareness. The counselor further challenged and encouraged me to take risks and move out of my comfort zone in being more direct, interactive, and even confrontational if it would enhance my growth and benefit the relationships.

I believe that the change in me was first seen and experienced in my role as pastor. Some persons were not used to my directness and clarity in what I thought and felt, how I approached them, and my assertiveness. With my children, I too was more open, honest, and direct, especially sharing my feelings and thoughts. I became more emotionally expressive and responsive, especially letting them know that I loved them. I have further become more intentional in sharing my life experiences with them when appropriate. Of course, I don't think they have been all that eager to hear of my experiences, but they do listen. My counseling experiences have been a significant catalyst for my personal growth at key points in my life.

RECOMMENDATIONS FOR COUNSELORS

Honoring the diversity among Black fathers

There is great diversity within and among Black people, and it is important for any counselor to get to know any Black fathers clients for the unique people we are. This includes understanding the intersectionality of his various identities and the salience of those identities and their influence on the client's worldview and lived experience. For example, for a counselor working with me, they would have to understand that I am a Black, male, Pentecostal Christian, and Baby Boomer in age, all of which influence how I see the world, the values I have, and how I interface with the world. As a child growing up the 1960s and one who vividly remembers James Brown singing "I'm Black and I'm Proud," I have a different view of the world today and much anger toward today's racist and xenophobic society than maybe a Black father born in the 1980s. While that same counselor may have another client with those same primary identities as me, there will be significant differences between myself and that client based on our education levels, areas of privilege, and our lived experiences. Counselors must acknowledge and honor the diversity among Black fathers.

In order to effectively work with Black fathers, counselors must take seriously the counseling profession's ethical mandate on multicultural competency. This means that a counselor possesses such self-awareness, knowledge, and skills to effectively form a counseling relationship with a client, who will be different than the counselor, and the counselor is able to address issues/concerns surrounding race, ethnicity, and the client's other salient identities, which will enhance the client's wellness, growth, and development. In working with Black fathers, this requires the counselor to be comfortable in talking about race and racism, especially in today's racial climate. In addition to multicultural competence, it may be important for counselors to possess spiritual competencies in working with Black fathers, who may see themselves as religious, spiritual, or spiritual and religious. Historically, Black people have used religion and spirituality as coping mechanisms against the negative effects of racism, which may or may not be true with today's Black fathers (Boyd-Franklin, 2010). Therefore, it is important for counselors to understand if and how a client's spirituality/religion may enhance well-being, contribute to client problems, and/or exacerbate symptoms (ASERVIC, 2009). For example, a Black father may believe that the Bible mandates him to beat his children with a belt, which has gotten the father in trouble with a child protection agency and now he has been mandated to counseling. The counselor may have to address the father's religious belief behind his behavior. Both multicultural and spiritual competencies will benefit counselors in working with Black fathers.

Addressing stigma

The issue of stigma associated with mental illness is prevalent not only in our society but also within Black communities (Heath, 2017). As counselors, we must find ways to combat the stigma for all persons which prevents them from seeking counseling. While Black men may not seek counseling in significant numbers, it might be worthwhile to consider alternative ways to offer counseling and support to Black fathers. For example, group counseling may be an option with potential clients seeing that they are not alone and meeting other Black fathers. Counselors can offer parenting workshops to equip and empower Black fathers. Offering counseling and such creative programming in a community setting, such as a Black church, may be appealing to Black fathers. With the Black Church's historical presence and service within Black communities (Lincoln & Mamiya, 1990), counselors may want to explore partnerships with Black churches to offer innovative programs to Black fathers.

CONCLUSION

Emerging adolescence represents a turbulent time of physical, social, and emotional growth for young people who are forming an ego identity and finding their place in the world. As young people in this Generation Z are reporting, they are experiencing significant stressors which are affecting their well-being and manifesting in negative mental health outcomes, such as anxiety and depression. Black fathers can be a stabilizing presence for their adolescent children during these years by affirming their ethnic identity, supporting their identify exploration, teaching them the realities of being Black in the world, providing wisdom to navigate the world of adult relationships, and providing a safe, nurturing, hospitable space to learn, heal, and grow from their lived experiences.

REFERENCES

American Counseling Association. (2014). *Code of ethics*. Alexandria, VA: Author.

Association for Spiritual, Ethical, and Religious Values in Counseling. (2009). Competencies for integrating spirituality into counseling. Retrieved from http://www.aservic.org/ resources/spiritual-competencies/.

Bang, H. (2015). African American undergraduate students' wisdom and ego-identity development: Effects of age, gender, self-esteem, and resilience. *Journal of Black Psychology*, *41*(2), 95–120.

Boyd-Franklin, N. (2010). Incorporating spirituality and religion into the treatment of African American clients. *The Counseling Psychologist*, *38*(7), 976–1000.

Brokaw, T. (2014). Tom Brokaw explains the origins of the greatest generation. Retrieved from https://www.nbcnews.com/video/tom-brokaw-explains-the-origins-of-the-greatest-generation-273640003752.

Desilver, D. (2019). The concerns and challenges of being a U.S. teen: What the data show. Pew Research Center. Retrieved from https://www.pewresearch.org/fact-tank/2019/02/26/the-concerns-and-challenges-of-being-a-u-s-teen-what-the-data-show/.

Dimock, M. (2019). Defining generations: Where Millennials end and Generation Z begins. Pew Research Center. Retrieved from https://www.pewresearch.org/fact-tank/2019/01/17/where-millennials-end-and-generation-z-begins/.

Erikson, E. H. (1963). *Childhood and society*. New York, NY: W. W. Norton & Company.

Erikson, E. H. (1968). *Identity: Youth and crisis*. New York, NY: W. W. Norton & Company.

Fry, R., & Parker, K. (2018). Early benchmarks show 'post-millennials' on track to be most diverse, best-educated generation yet. Pew Research Center. Retrieved from https://www.pewsocialtrends.org/2018/11/15/early-benchmarks-show-post-millennials-on-track-to-be-most-diverse-best-educated-generation-yet/.

Geiger, A. W., & Davis, L. (2019). A growing number of American teenagers – particularly girls – are facing depression. Pew Research Center. Retrieved from https://www.pewresearch.org/fact-tank/2019/07/12/a-growing-number-of-american-teenagers-particularly-girls-are-facing-depression/.

Heath, S. (2017). Understanding stigma as a mental healthcare barrier. Retrieved from https://patientengagementhit.com/news/understanding-stigma-as-a-mental-healthcare-barrier?utm_content=b1281c3eaa9e820f79ecee0fe1311937&utm_campaign=MHD%25206%252F8%252F17&utm_source=Robly.com&utm_medi.

Hettler, W. (1976). Six dimensions of wellness model. National Institute of Wellness. Retrieved from https://cdn.ymaws.com/www.nationalwellness.org/resource/resmgr/pdfs/SixDimensionsFactSheet.pdf.

Horowitz, J. M., & Graf, N. (2019). Most U.S. teens see anxiety and depression as a major problem among their peers. Pew Research Center. Retrieved from https://www.pewsocialtrends.org/2019/02/20/most-u-s-teens-see-anxiety-and-depression-as-a-major-problem-among-their-peers/.

Kelly, M. (2005). *The seven levels of intimacy: The art of loving and the joy of being loved*. New York: Fireside.

Kottler, J. A. (2010). *On being a therapist*. San Francisco, CA: Jossey-Bass.

Lewis, S. (2019). The racial bias built into photography. *New York Times*, April 25, 2019. New York: New York Times.

Lincoln, C. E., & Mamiya, L. H. (1990). *The Black church in the African American experience*. Durham, NC: Duke University Press.

Marcia, J. E. (1966). Development and validation of ego-identity status. *Journal of Personality and Social Psychology*, *3*(5), 551–558.

Nouwen, H. J. (1975). *Reaching out: The three movements of the spiritual life*. New York: Doubleday.

Parrott, L., & Parrott, L. (2015). *Saving your marriage before it starts: Seven questions to ask before – and after – you marry*. Grand Rapids, MI: Zondervan.

Roscoe, L. J. (2009). Wellness: A review of theory and measurement for counselors. *Journal of Counseling and Development*, *87*, 216–226.

St. Louis, G. R., & Liem, J. H. (2005). Ego identity, ethnic identity, and the psychosocial well-being of ethnic minority and majority college students. *Identity: An International Journal of Theory and Research*, *5*(3), 227–246.

Staples, B. (2019). How blackface feeds White supremacy. *New York Times*, March 31, 2019. New York: New York Times.

Sue, D. W., Nadal, K. L., Capodilupo, C. M., Lin, A. I., Torino, G. C., & Rivera, D. P. (2008). Racial microaggressions against Black Americans: Implications for counseling. *Journal of Counseling & Development*, *86*, 330–338.

Tynes, B. M., Umana-Taylor, A. J., Rose, C. A., Lin, J., & Anderson, C. J. (2012). Online racial discrimination and the protective function of ethnic identity and self-esteem for African American adolescents. *Developmental Psychology*, *48*(2), 343–355.

CHAPTER EIGHT

Supporting Adolescent Mental Health

MICHAEL D. HANNON, PHD, LAC, NCC

FATHER PROFILE

Michael Hannon has been married to LaChan since August 2000 and they have two children. Nile, his daughter, is 18. Avery, his son, is 16. Since 2000, Michael has served in a range of counseling roles beginning in student affairs, school counseling, and clinical mental health counseling. He has a doctoral degree (PhD) in counselor education and supervision and is an associate professor in the counseling program at Montclair State University in New Jersey.

BIGGEST INFLUENCES ON MY FATHERING

My father has and continues to have the biggest influence on my fathering. I would describe my relationship with my dad as healthy and continuing to evolve. He, my mom, and our extended family and community provided for my sisters and me opportunities and experiences that privileged us in many ways. My dad was and is accessible, engaged, and has always actively loved me. Looking back, I can acknowledge—now—how he has transformed emotionally throughout my life. He is a private and guarded man who, over time, actively matched his, "I love you" words with deep hugs and kisses on my cheek. I remember this especially as a teenager, and I was usually cool with it. I appreciated it then and to this day, I greet him with a hug and kiss most times when I see him. I have also deeply benefitted from diverse fathering examples through my many uncles (by blood and by marriage), my grandfathers, my father-in-law, soccer and wrestling coaches, pastors and friends of faith, and my beloved college friends and fraternity brothers. However, my dad—by far—has been the biggest influence on my fathering.

While he exhibits a wider range of emotional variability now, the default posture for my dad is as a quiet observer. If you don't know him, it can sometimes present as judgmental but I know he's not judging anyone. He's become increasingly aware of this, too. I notice how his posture changes so that his body language matches his verbal language, especially in new spaces. My family has a running joke about this. My dad and I have been told that we look mad or upset, when that's actually the least accurate description about our mood. When this happens, LaChan will gently ask, "Hey, is everything ok? Is something wrong?" He or I have frequently responded saying that we are just fine. In response, she says, "Well, you need to tell your face, then!" This usually ends up with us laughing at ourselves. And smiling more.

My dad has an incredible work ethic and I know he has always worked hard to provide for us financially; I don't ever remember needing for anything. If we did, my parents shielded me from that. I remember always having a full belly, being able to go shopping for kicks and gear when I need them, and the family car(s) were pretty functional. But, to hear my parents tell it, they'd remind me that—for a very specific time—those meals were inexpensive (lots of pasta, deli meats, etc.), gear and shoes were bought from the local marketplace, and when the car is called "The Brown Bomb" by friends and family, it was just that: functional. For me, this translated into genuinely believing my dad knew everything. Here's a testament to who I thought my dad was until I was about 12 years old.

My family has always celebrated Christmas. On this particular Christmas, my parents bought the family our first video cassette recorder, or VCR. We were excited. My dad just got a membership card at the local, mom and pop video rental store in the next town over from ours; I guess this was the precursor to chains like Blockbuster. Anyway, as we wanted to get the VCR set up to the family television, my dad seemed frustrated. He was having trouble interpreting the directions.

At one point, I (insensitively) asked him, "Dad, how come you don't know how to put this together?" He sharply replied, "Michael, I don't know everything!"

Mind. Officially. Blown. This took some reconciling for me because my dad was my personal superhero. At 46 years old, I can still attest that he's my superhero, flaws and all. This was and is particularly important for me as I consider my own fathering practices, strengths, insecurities, and limitations. I continue to learn that it is fine to not know everything. I have learned from my father—and otherfathers—that many if not most mistakes are recoverable, even in a horribly anti-Black world. However, I'd be lying if I said I was assured of this notion of being able to make mistakes when my family confronted one of our most significant challenges.

CONFRONTING SYMPTOMS OF DEPRESSION AND ANXIETY—DURING AND AFTER CRISIS

It was August 2018 and I was excited at the prospect of going overseas. I was invited to participate in a research symposium at Oxford University with about 15 other mental health professionals and researchers from around the world. Our agenda included learning from each other about our professional/research interests and how mental health services were administered in each of our respective countries and local communities. I was there to discuss my research—and my lived experience—on Black fathers of students with autism. I wanted to share what I've learned from interviewing so many fathers of children with developmental differences about what they recommended for schools and other agencies to support fathers more effectively engage them more successfully. It was an opportunity that excited me because I realized how privileged I was to even go. And learn. And share. This was big shit to me. Like, real big.

The trip was special for another reason, too. My daughter, Nile, was supposed to join me in London after my research conference. We were going to spend the following week touring London and then visiting Black Paris. It was an early 16th birthday gift, and LaChan and I were in a position to give it to her. Things would go very differently in the two days leading up to the trip, though.

On what seemed a typical afternoon on my way to get my son, Avery, from his summer theatre camp, Nile told me she needed to go to the hospital. She'd been resting all day after leaving her volunteer site early from being sick.

> [annoyed and dismissively I said] "For what?"
> "I took too much medicine."
>
> "Pain reliever? [then I begin to piece it together … she has my undivided attention] How much did you take?"
>
> "15" [her eyes begin to tear up]
>
> "When? When did you take them?"
>
> "At 10 this morning." [It's 2:30 PM and now I know why she's been throwing up all day. I'm almost panicking but calm enough to say firmly]
>
> "Put your shit on. We've got to go to the hospital."

This experience was excruciating—and healing—in a number of ways. It required Nile to get more intensive counseling support. She was hospitalized for close to two weeks. Thereafter, she had intensive outpatient counseling services for another month. And she still sees her therapist at least once a week. Nile is being treated for anxiety and depression.

Prior to this crisis—and opportunity—my fathering of Nile was imbalanced. Did I spend time with her? Sure. We especially enjoy going to the movies and going out to eat. Nile LOVES to eat out. Occasionally, I would invade the space with her and friends or jokingly crawl in her bed as she attempted to rest on a Saturday morning.

It would always make me proud to hear her share her opinions. Nile has strong social justice convictions and I always appreciate talking about current events with her and how our highly politicized times translate into our daily lives.

But, I mistakenly allowed her to develop habits as a teenager that I have as an adult. This typically came in the form of spending time alone. I would let her spend alone time in her room to work or to browse her computer because I often work alone in my home office.

Nile and I are similar. While we enjoy people's company, we don't often seek it. This yields significant amounts of isolated time unless we have people in our lives to get us up and out. I was allowing Nile to act like me in ways that she wasn't ready to handle responsibly or maturely. We both have HIGH FEELINGS quotients and sometimes those feelings can be hard to manage.

COUNSELING SUPPORT FOR US

Our experience required us to get family counseling, LaChan and I to get couples counseling, and for me to get individual counseling. That requires a lot of talking. And work. It was especially important for me to find Black counselors to work with us once we were able to choose our service providers. The counselors working with us are all Black women who understand and appreciate the value we place on our cultural and familial norms, our faith, our language, and how we interpret the world around us filtered through our Blackness.

In family counseling we've been learning strategies to check in more frequently with each other and to be clearer about how we are all feeling. Simple techniques that many counselors and teachers use frequently, like scaling (e.g., "On a scale of 1 to 10, how you rate your nervousness?), now have a different and more important meaning and context. We are now spending more time in the same space and less time separated. We are working harder to accurately interpret each other's words and behaviors to better support each other. This often requires more questions, more answers, but ultimately, more engagement. Our family therapists have been using Dialectical Behavioral Therapy (DBT) with us toward these goals. There has been homework, increased attention to emotional intelligence and emotion regulation, learning more about how I can support Nile by asking her more pointed questions and investing more time with her.

In couples and individual counseling, I'm still learning to not be as guarded. This comes by way of me (genuinely) laughing more and showing a much broader range of emotions to my family. I'm also trying to be honest and admit—openly and not defensively—there are things I just don't know; I'm learning that it is admirable and necessary to ask for help.

I am learning that fathering my daughter requires support that is different than the kind I attempt to give Avery. Fathering Nile requires me to learn even more about myself. I'm learning that I don't like failing, or even the perception that I failed. And when I do believe I've failed, I most frequently blame myself and harbor guilt as a result. Nile is similar to me, in that way. Ultimately, I am learning that Nile values my time and experiences with me, versus things and assets I can give her.

RECOMMENDATIONS FOR COUNSELORS WORKING WITH BLACK FATHERS

Educate and Be Educated. Black fathers raising children who need specific mental health support can fall victim to being questioning or even dismissive of diagnoses. This questioning can be for a number of reasons, many times based on stereotypes about the reality of mental wellness and illness and the genuine distrust Black and other historically marginalized people have for systems of care. Vontress and Epp (1997) and Whaley (2001) have written extensively about historical hostility, or "the pattern of responses that many African-Americans exhibit, which may stem from their prolonged subjection to inferior treatment in American society"(p. 170) and cultural mistrust, which is a disposition Black people have toward White Americans in response to historical and contemporary experiences of oppression.

I would encourage counselors to educate Black fathers—as needed—on the counseling process (e.g., how sessions can look and feel; how time can be spent during session) and on what can help support their children's wellness, especially in ways that will be new and unfamiliar. Many Black fathers parent in ways they've been parented. Likewise, I can't understate the value of demonstrating cultural humility to assist with providing culturally responsive counseling support. My friend and colleague and I wrote about making sure to refrain from reducing Black male clients to their presenting issues or problems (Hannon & Vereen, 2016). This applies especially now, with counselors encouraged to be clinically and genuinely curious about and willing to learn from their Black father clients' experiences and knowledge.

Connect. I would also encourage counselors working with Black fathers of children with specific mental health needs to advocate for them connecting with other (Black) fathers. Men, in general, seem to value connecting with other men with shared lived experiences. The group counseling tenet of universality – or the experience of not being alone in a lived experience - can be deeply valuable for Black fathers as they navigate their manhood while supporting their children's mental health and wellness.

Celebrate. American fathers, and Black fathers included, can be very performance driven. As counselors work with Black fathers toward goals, I encourage counselors to celebrate those achievements as a way to reinforce the value of counseling work. Helping Black fathers learn to negotiate their children's needs while possibly being in environments that may not readily understand or accept mental health those needs can be challenging. All goals achieved are worth the acknowledgement and celebration.

REFERENCES

Hannon, M. D., & Vereen, L. G. (2016). Irreducibility of Black male clients: Considerations for culturally competent counseling. *Journal of Humanistic Counseling*, *55*, 234–245. DOI: 10.1002/johc.12036.

Vontress, C. E., & Epp, L. (1997). Historical hostility in the African-American client: Implications for counseling. *Journal of Multicultural Counseling and Development*, *25*, 170–184.

Whaley, A. L. (2001). Cultural mistrust and mental health services for African-Americans: A review and meta-analysis. *The Counseling Psychologist*, *29*, 513–531.

CHAPTER NINE

Fathering Adolescents for Post-secondary Success

RODNEY N. WEST, MA

FATHER PROFILE

Rodney West has been married to Nicole Jeter West since 2000 and they have three children. Their son Xavier is 15 years old; son Tyler is 12; and their daughter Sydney is eight years old. Rodney worked in the financial industry for 15 years as a business analyst and project manager before becoming a professional school counselor in 2018. Rodney is a school counselor at Piscataway High School in New Jersey, where approximately 2200 students attend.

BIGGEST INFLUENCES ON FATHERING

I have been very fortunate to be surrounded by many men who have had a great influence on my ability to father. Although most have been positive influences, there have been a few who have taught me to be a better father by showing me what not to do. First, I have learned that being an absent father often has little to do with locale. Fathers can be physically present, but mentally and emotionally absent. In many conversations with my father, he often expressed to me that although he lived in the same house with my grandfather, they were very distant from each other. They spoke only when my grandfather was doling out punishment. My father and his siblings were rarely offered a "congratulations!" or a "good job!"

My dad told me that on some days, his dad may not even say hello.

I often saw a similar dearth of communication in the relationships that my friends had with their fathers. Their fathers worked and provided for their families, but did not have much of an emotional connection with their children. They did not converse with their children nor their children's friends; they did not attend any school-related events. They may attend athletic events, usually to drink beer in the parking lot and to gloat about their children's on-field accomplishments. As with my grandfather, my friends' fathers made their presence felt when there was a need for lectures and/or consequences. I can only assume that these fathers believed that as long as they provided financially, they did not have to do nor be anything else. As long as they provided a place to live and sleep, put food on the table and clothes on their children's backs, their mission was accomplished. Maybe they believed that providing these material necessities equaled fatherhood. Maybe they believed emotional support and verbal encouragement were not necessities.

This is why I believe that location—while helpful in fathering—is not necessary for good fathering.

One can be supportive without being in the same space. As a school counselor, I work with students whose fathers are not physically around. I also work with students whose fathers are physically around, yet those students wish they weren't. The result is the same: anger, frustration, disappointment, emotional distance.

Secondly, the ability to make financial contributions do not make men good fathers. I have learned that paying child-support or giving money to children is not a substitute for anything in the child-rearing process. It appeared to me that financial support was a Band-Aid that would temporarily cover the wound left by many fathers' disconnection or emotional absence. That new pair of sneakers feels great until the child realizes that his father is not coming to see his first game. Or his second game. I have friends and relatives who call it "providing" when they buy material items or send money. When that child needs something that money cannot buy—support, attention, encouragement, a voice of calm—he will not call his father.

This is not an indictment of fathers who do not live with their children, nor is it an implication that fathers with extraordinary responsibilities outside the home cannot be good fathers. Those men can be great fathers—and a lot of them are—if they are providing what their children need. Children's needs are more than material things.

On the other hand, I did have positive fatherly influences in my life who helped me become a better father. My father, Ronald West, has been the best example and has made the greatest impact on my ability to father. Just as I learned what not to do from others around me, my father was shown the same by his own father. My father was the fifth of six children. They were raised in a two-bedroom row house in North Philadelphia. As mentioned, my father and his brothers and sister did not have much of a relationship with their father. My father graduated from Ben Franklin High School and went on to Lincoln University with the intention of never going back to Philly. He graduated from Lincoln and moved to New Jersey with one suitcase and no money. Still refusing to move back to Philly, he rented a room at the YMCA in New Brunswick, NJ. He landed a job as a line supervisor at the Johnson and Johnson factory where he met my mother.

Amongst so many memories about my childhood, what I remember the most is that my father was always there; he was always present. As children, my sister played softball and danced, my brother was a boy scout and played baseball, while I played football, basketball, and baseball. My father was at every practice, every game, every parent meeting, and every awards ceremony for each of us. He was my brother's den leader; he volunteered as my baseball coach (having never played the game himself); he attended almost all of my Pop Warner football practices, either as a volunteer in some capacity or as a proud father. And he attended almost every game of every sport that I ever played. When a friend needed a ride home from practice, he automatically asked me because he knew my father was coming.

At the time, I did not pay attention to how meaningful this was. For me, this was normal; my friends seemed to appreciate it more than I did.

As we got older and talked about past events, I then began to notice how often my father was present—both physically and emotionally—as compared to some of their fathers. I have a childhood friend who went on to play Division I football in the ACC; yet his father never saw him play.

There were times when my father could not attend some events, but there was always a reason—working late, church event, or being sick. He never missed anything because he "didn't feel like it" and I knew—without doubt—that my siblings and I were his priority. One day during my teenage years, my father told me (without prompting) how and why he felt the need to be at everything. He explained that it was because his father never did anything with him or for him, and he remembers how that made him feel.

He felt dismissed and disregarded, as if he didn't matter. He wanted to be certain that his kids never felt that way, and they knew that he cared.

Whenever we were together, there was always conversation about sports, girls, or life. During my teenage years, the conversations became more mature as he helped me sort out my battles with peer pressure, relationships, and "growing up too fast." He constantly shared stories about his childhood and the things he saw, with the intent of helping me to avoid some of the mistakes he made. He was always emotionally available, which increased his desire to be physically available.

When Nicole was pregnant with our first child, I told my father that I was scared. I wasn't the worst child; but I was far from the best. It felt hypocritical to chastise my son if/when he does some of the same things that I did. Pop said something that I have never forgotten. He said,

"Nobody said you will be perfect. To be a good father, all you have to do is care. If you care, you will do your best to do the right thing. You won't always be right, but you will always try your best."

This advice, as well as all of the stories that he shared throughout my life would guide my parenting and would inspire me to be a caring, available, and emotionally present Black father.

FATHERING TEENAGERS

Being the father of a teenager is more difficult than one may think. That is not to say that it is more difficult than being the parent of a pre-teen; but there are different challenges. In 2011, Nicole and I had the fortune of becoming the legal guardians of two of Nicole's teenage cousins due to some family issues. A 17-year-old boy and a 15-year-old girl came to live with us until they finished high school. They moved to New Jersey from Florida, and Nicole and I had not seen them in years. At the time, Xavier was seven years old and Tyler was four; the boys never met them. And, Nicole was pregnant with Sydney.

Over the first few weeks that they lived with us, we discovered that we knew nothing about parenting teenagers.

We also felt like becoming effective parents of teenagers after a lifetime of habits, routines, and expectations have already been established was damn near impossible.

We took the first few months to get to know each other—tendencies, regimens, likes, and dislikes—before considering what things needed to remain and what changes needed to be made. Their prior upbringing was nothing like what we had begun to establish for our own kids. Their previous family dynamic allowed them to do as they pleased. The girl was forced to be more of an adult—like a parentified child—taking care of her older brother, and their young sister (she did not move in with us). Consequently, she thought she was an adult, and could do and say whatever she wanted. The boy did nothing, nor did he know how. He ate, slept, and watched television. Nicole and I agreed that those habits had to be changed for their own benefit, but we didn't know how to change them.

We often had to check ourselves, being mindful that they are not used to having two parents, nor having to follow rules set by someone other than themselves.

We understood and agreed that their transition to being members of a nuclear family could not be immediate, and it would not be seamless. There were several conversations and several arguments amongst all of us. There were many tense situations as the girl wanted to leave on multiple occasions, and I was ready to oblige most of those times. Later, while a counseling student and learning the influence of parenting, I realized that a lot of their impulsive reactions were, in part, a reflection of the relationships they had with their parents. Their father was physically absent, while their mother was emotionally detached. In many ways, they were forced to raise themselves. We were literally living with teenagers who were sent mixed messages all the time! They enjoyed yet resented the idea of having parents. They appreciated coming home to a peaceful environment and having someone to help them with their growth and development and encourage them when things went well. However, they did not like the idea of having to follow rules, meet sometimes challenging expectations, and be confronted when those rules were broken or expectations not met.

Those two and a half years were difficult, but they were a great learning experience in assertiveness, patience, listening, and parenting in general. We learned that as parents of teens one has to manage the many dimensions of the teenage experience: hormones, attitudes, peer pressure, curiosity, and/or experimentation with drugs, alcohol, sex, and sexual orientation. In addition, it feels like technology compounds every issue. Parents have to contend with their teenagers having access to the entire world in their pockets in the form of a smartphone.

Of course YouTube, Instagram, and TikTok can tell them more than we can!

We learned that the relationship between parents and children can have direct and lasting impacts on children's emotional development. Parents' emotional distance can negatively affect their children's personality and ability to socially interact. We learned that although issues (behavioral, verbal, academic) must be addressed with immediacy, the approach is not absolute. As teens have begun to develop their own personalities, I believe that the imposed discipline can be more impactful depending on its delivery. For example, yelling at someone who is just going to cry may not be as effective as having a stern conversation. When Nicole's cousins moved in with us my mentality (and probably disposition) reflected probably something my grandfather might say: "It's my house, my rules!" Throughout that time and when Xavier reached his teens, I learned to keep the same mindset, but modify my delivery to be more effective.

We also learned that there is a delicate balance to creating an environment that is safe for everyone. As parents of teenagers, we had to learn how to give them space to grow, yet help keep them accountable so they would be successful whenever they left us. As a counselor in the same high school that my son attends, I do my best to let Xavier enjoy his time as a teenager in high school; but he knows that I'm there. Not as a disciplinarian (although I will if I have to), but as a guide to help him both mitigate and learn from mistakes. It is a similar concept at home—let him be a teenager and give him the space to make choices, have fun, make mistakes, and learn from it all; he also knows that I am here, to advise, support, and challenge.

And regulate, when necessary.

RECOMMENDATIONS FOR COUNSELORS

Being thrown into the middle of raising teenagers, I wish I had someone to talk to during that time. My friends did not have teenage children. Our parents' old school mentality and approach were often ineffective. Our lack of parenting knowledge caused more tension in our home than we ever had before as we had to develop the skills to parent teenagers. I definitely could have benefitted from individual counseling, and my family would definitely have benefited from couples or family counseling. However, having that experience has made the second attempt at parenting teenagers easier to manage. Those two and a half years gave me some foresight in preparing for Xavier's teenage years.

Most fathers will not have the same opportunity. Hindsight is always twenty-twenty; football fans call this being a Monday morning quarterback. For counselors working with Black fathers of teenagers, I ask counselors to:

1. Encourage Black fathers to be honest and vulnerable by showing their teenagers they care. Simple, but undervalued skills like active listening and asking questions go a long way with teenagers. Counselors know how valuable it is for anyone—especially teenagers—to feel heard and affirmed.
2. Encourage Black fathers to be flexible as they learn about their teenagers. Every teenager will be different and fathers—like all parents—can develop expectations about who they think their children should be. If or when those expectations aren't realized, the fathers may feel like they have experienced a loss. This flexibility will help them support their teenagers in what can be a really challenging time in life.
3. Remind Black fathers that with support, their children can overcome challenges. Teenagers will make mistakes. And the stakes are higher for Black children's mistakes. However, reminding Black fathers that with support of the community, and the trust of their teenagers, they can own

and redeem their mistakes. Counselors are in a unique position to help Black fathers help their teens understand their mistakes and assist with correcting them.

4. Support Black fathers as they guide their teens into adulthood with their own identities. Counselors might realize that Black fathers—like many parents—might be inclined to mold their teens into who they want them to be. However, a healthy (even while still developing) identity will be much more helpful and healthy for teenagers than becoming who their fathers want them to become. Counselors are aware of how valuable encouraging a solid sense of personal and racial identity can be for teenagers and young adults.

Black fathering can be intimidating, pressure-filled, and outright scary because of things like peer pressure and technology. It is important for our teenagers to know that their Black fathers are not just an entity, but we are Black men who have an intimate and dedicated stake in their growth, development, and success. Being a good Black father takes time, effort, and commitment. Most importantly, like my father told me, it takes the willingness to care.

CHAPTER TEN

Black Adult Children on Their Black Fathers: A Retrospective

GELAWDIYOS M. HAILE, PHD, AMBER S. HALEY, PHD, AMBER R. NORMAN, PHD, S. KENT BUTLER, PHD

BLACK FATHERS' MENTAL HEALTH

What is a father? And what does it mean to be a Black father in America? Throughout the course of time, Black men and fathers have consistently shown their ability to persevere and be resilient in the face of structural and institutional racism. They demonstrate a commitment to assume their responsibilities as fathers, challenging the dominant racist trope about absentee Black fathers. This chapter, in comparison to others, is a composite of our collective reflections about our fathers now that we are adults at different points in our lives. Our experiences are similar and different in many ways. However, the beauty of sharing this with you is the opportunity to share what we know about how our Black fathers have cared for us in our adulthood in all of its beauty, complexity, and challenge. Thank you for engaging with us on this narrative journey.

The ways fathers influence their adult children take on multiple forms. Much of the influence happens before the child leaves the home (i.e., from childhood to early adulthood). For instance, fathers have the opportunity to model positive masculinity to their children (Roberts-Douglass & Curtis-Boles, 2013). And research has told us that the bond between fathers and sons can influence the sons' attachment style during adulthood (Willis & Clark, 2009). For Black young adults, their fathers play a role in the form of guidance, support, and counsel (Peart, Pungello, Campbell, & Richey, 2006). It goes without saying that Black fathers and father figures are "jacks of all trades," many times providing the kind of support that others might seek from professional counselors. For example, counseling support may not be accessible or affordable for many Black families. And, for the families for whom it is affordable, there could be a legitimate and tangible lack of trust in the healthcare system. Black families would be more likely to seek counseling and mental health support from their faith leaders (e.g., pastors, Imams, etc.) than from professional counselors.

Our relationships with our fathers are diverse. Some of us would describe our relationships with our fathers as deeply engaged, estranged, or even nonexistent. Disclosing this much is even a challenge. Our fathers, admittedly, have had varying levels of interactions with us across our lives. Some of us maintain meaningful, deep, and mutually beneficial relationships with our fathers as adults. And some of us have been disassociated from our fathers due to real issues like age difference, divorce, or distance that can absolutely strain father–child relationships, even when those children are adults. What follows is our reporting of an informal interview with one of our Black fathers discussing how he supports his adult child, with insights on the type of mental health support that would be helpful for him. The interview integrates concepts from Bill Hettler's (1976) Six Dimensions of Wellness with follow-up questions to identify the father's level of involvement in emotional, spiritual, occupational, intellectual, physical, and social areas domains of his adult child's life. Here are some highlights from the interview.

Our interviewee told us that **he emotionally supported his child by providing unconditional love, respect, and psychological and emotional support. His spiritual support included reminding his adult child of her religious values and environments where those values were honored and affirmed. The father we interviewed spoke in very clear terms about the occupational support he has tried to provide his adult child. He shared that he has consistently encouraged an appreciation for the value of tangible and intangible possessions. It has also been important to provide advice and—when necessary—financial assistance. Intellectually, this father's support has come in the form of supporting his adult child's educational pursuits and growth in career choices. Physically, he has encouraged his adult child to remain active, have fun, and live a balanced life. In the social dimension, this father advised his child to set boundaries, be kind always, and work hard to maintain healthy relationships.** Most importantly, when it comes to decision-making and their children's independence, fathers asserted that they respected their children's independence and trusted their ability to make decisions for themselves. Here are direct quotes from our interviewed father about supporting his adult child, with our insights and inferences in italics when necessary.

WHAT DOES IT MEAN TO BE A FATHER AND HOW IS YOUR ROLE AS A FATHER INFLUENCED BY YOUR CULTURAL BACKGROUND?

A father means that I am responsible for the safety, well-being, nourishment, and the spiritual and emotional growth of my children because I love them and want the best for them.

My role as a father is influenced by my cultural background in the sense that I am always being made aware of the stigmas and stereotypes of my culture which makes me prepare my children for the society they may face. My culture has also been interwoven with military culture, so I have been able to learn from positive and negative role models. I prepare my children by teaching them the importance of a good education and that there is not much room for failure in this world. You can't waste time by not knowing; you have to be decisive and work harder than the perceived standard at whatever you want in life because everyone does not have the same starting line in this race. Train your mind to expect the best, because when you don't get it, it will be motivation to get what you feel is rightfully yours. When you fail, it is always your fault. Find out what you could have done better instead of blaming someone else for your failure. This showcases boldly the actions of a father who believes in tough love. This type of parenting could cause children to rebel and seek nurturance elsewhere. *A culturally attuned counselor would be a positive change for a socially distanced father that parents in this manner. It would behoove counselors to understand the influences of this Black father's attitudes about failure and what causes it. Counselors who demonstrate empathy regarding the immense pressure Black men and fathers experienced to conform and comport when given opportunities for economic mobility can perhaps provide insight to this perspective.*

WHAT SUPPORT SYSTEMS ARE IN PLACE FOR YOU PARENTING AN ADULT CHILD AND WHAT SUPPORT SYSTEMS DO YOU PROVIDE FOR YOUR ADULT CHILD?

My support system is my relationship with God and His guidance and my willingness to continue to grow spiritually, personally, and professionally. It is the foundation of my being. God's word has taught me that love is a verb; you love your neighbor by how you behave toward them regardless of how they behave toward you. Godly character teaches behavior that endures and withstands the test of time contrary to how we normally would react out of fear when faced with controversy. It teaches to remain hopeful when it appears that no hope is in sight.

It is how I remain positive no matter what the situation looks like. *This Black father's reliance on his Christian faith provides a window into how he is able to sustain himself and support his family in a racist and unsupportive world. This Black father's faith is a protective factor that can be acknowledged and highlighted in a counseling relationship.*

I provide support systems for my adult child that shows a life example of how sticking to something long enough will pay off but revealing my vulnerabilities to express the fact that everything is a process and takes hard work and to never stop trying to get things right. Nothing is by chance. I provide advice when asked (the hard truth that only a father can give). I provide financial support as a last resort to teach my child that there are no safety nets in life; you will pay for the consequences of your decisions and indecisions. *Counselors working with this Black father can highlight how he demonstrates and models his resilience in an anti-Black world and challenge him to demonstrate empathy and the importance of deep relationships to convey that while there are no safety nets, his children can count on support and acceptance unconditionally from him.*

The responses above provide us insight about the complexity of Black fatherhood and they demonstrate why counselors can benefit from a more robust research base on Black fathers. Black men and fathers confront unique adversities over the lifespan that may have adverse influences on their mental well-being (Tsuchiya, Qian, Thomas, Loney, & Caldwell, 2018; Watkins, 2012). Coupled with these challenges is the reality that Black people, in general, and Black men, in particular, seek mental health services less frequently than people from other racial groups (Cheng & Robinson, 2013).

BLACK FATHERS AND THEIR SUPPORT FOR FINANCIAL LITERACY AND CAREER STABILITY

Given our collective experiences and the responses from our interviewee, we know our fathers desired for us to have financial literacy and experience career stability. Beyond our general happiness, our fathers' desire for us to be financial stable is among their strongest desires. Counselors working with Black fathers of adult children should be attuned to this desire for their children as an indicator of their own fathering success and effectiveness. Further, counselors working with Black father clients need to understand and be culturally responsive to how unemployment impacts Black communities. According to the United States Department of Labor Statistics, the unemployment rate for Black or African Americans 16 years old or over has decreased from a high of 16.1% in December 2009 to 6% as of June 2019 (U.S. Bureau of Labor Statistics, 2019a). It may be worth noting that this decline in Black or African American unemployment rates largely coincide with the presidency of Barack Obama from January 20, 2009 until January 20, 2017. President Obama's first term was marked by action addressing the global financial crisis including a major stimulus package, partial extension of tax cuts, and a financial regulation reform bill. Despite these improvements, Black or African American unemployment rates are still twice as high as White unemployment rates in the U.S. (Wilson, 2019).

And then there is this thing called COVID

To compound the already disparaging rates of unemployment in Black communities, the *tridemic* of 2020, a term used to refer to the COVID-19 health, economic, and social justice crises in America, mark a significant turn in the unemployment and financial well-being of Black, Indigenous, and People of Color BIPOC (U.S. Bureau of Labor Statistics, 2020). From the month of March 2020 to present, there have been millions of Americans that have been negatively impacted by a disproportionate number of deaths by COVID-19 including co-morbidity of pre-existing conditions. This travesty also comes attached to alarming rates of unemployment, homelessness, and adult children and their children returning home due to these unforeseen economic, societal, and health crises (U.S. Bureau of Labor Statistics, 2020). Children spanning in age from early childhood through college age and adulthood have all been impacted by remote learning circumstances as schools across the country closed its doors and campuses in an attempt to curb the spread of the coronavirus. This mandate created a mass return of adult children across diverse financial means and stages of life home to live with their adult parents. For many of these Black adult children, this return home has caused a disruption to their work life, daily responsibilities, and feelings of independence.

Prior to the COVID 19 pandemic, research indicated a decline in young adults deciding to have children of their own and beginning a family, relative to that of their parents in previous generations. According to the National Center for Health Statistics, the United States' birth rate fell for a fifth consecutive year in 2019, bringing the lowest number of babies born in the U.S. to the lowest level it has been in 35 years (Centers for Disease Control and Prevention, 2020). Potential factors contributing to this decline in birth rate includes fewer teenage pregnancies and an increase of contraception use in the U.S. Also of impact is the lingering effects of the Great Recession, which has made it more difficult for individuals in their 20s and 30s to reach developmental milestones such as marriage, establishing a career, or buying a home—which have traditionally preceded starting a family (Holohan, 2020). This decline in young adults' ability to establish stability and financial security in their adult years has also affected the role and support African American fathers play in their adult children lives, as many adults are leaving home and still dependent on their parents for financial support.

Lastly, according to a report published by the TIAA Institute and the Global Financial Literacy Excellence Center, there is a significant gap in financial literacy among Black adults (TIAA Institute, 2020). The Personal Finance Index (P-Fin Index) is a measurement of U.S. adults' readiness to make sound financial decisions and examines financial literacy across eight areas: earning, consuming, saving, investing, borrowing, insuring, understanding risk, and gathering information (Thornton, 2019). *Financial Literacy and Wellness among African-Americans: New Insights from the Personal Finance (P-Fin) Index* reports that African Americans answered 38% of the Personal Finance (P-Fin) Index questions correctly compared with 55% among White adults , indicating a significant financial literacy gap (TIAA Institute). According to the report, a significant financial literacy gap exists in African American adults regardless of gender, age, income level, or degree of education and the head of the TIAA Institute asserted that it is imperative to continue shedding light on this disparity to better map a course for financial success (Thornton, 2019).

"Increasing efforts to promote research-based financial education in school and the workplace is one key solution for promoting financial well-being among African Americans" (Thornton, 2019). "Our research finds that African Americans tend to exhibit lower financial well-being than their White U.S. counterparts. Given the strong link between financial literacy and financial well-being, increased financial knowledge may lead to improved financial capability and behaviors" (Thornton, fifth section). It is reasonable to believe that an increase in financial literacy and generational wealth in African American adults may close the financial literacy gap between African Americans and other ethnic groups within the U.S. population, especially in comparison to their White counterparts, thereby increasing financial well-being within the African American community along with an ability to live independently as adult children, loved, but away from their fathers.

A bittersweet conclusion

Our interviewee stated something that resonates with the financial literacy information that we have provided. The father, like many we are sure, stated, "I taught my child that they should pursue careers they enjoy and careers that come easy to them because being in a career where there is a constant struggle will eventually cause burnout, lack of passion, and unfulfillment no matter how much money it provides." Our interests and passions influence our decisions. They provide keen insight, which may foster a life of excellence or render a life full of mediocrity. A strong fatherly role model raises their young child into adult children who are able to thrive under any circumstance. It is vital that Black fathers communicate with and teach their children important life lessons that build up character and resiliency. Looking back, an adult child may smile and say, because of him I am free, fiercely independent, and confident in my ability to persevere through any trial, tribulation, or triumph that happens upon my way. A true testament of a strong father figure is an adult child who was taught how to fish so that they could eat, feed, and teach these lessons for generations to come.

•

REFERENCES

Centers for Disease Control and Prevention. (2020). *National Center for Health Statistics*. https://www.cdc.gov/nchs/index.htm

Cheng, T. C., & Robinson, M. A. (2013). Factors leading African Americans and Black Caribbeans to use social work services for treating mental and substance use disorders. *Health & Social Work*, *38*(2), 99–109.

Economic Policy Institute. (n.d.). *EPI analysis of Bureau of Labor Statistics Local Area Unemployment Statistics (LAUS) data and Current Population Survey (CPS) data*. https://www.bls.gov/lau/

Hettler, B. (1976). The six dimensions of wellness. http://www.hettler.com/sixdimen.htm

Holohan, M. (2020, May 20). Birth rates in the US decline to lowest level in 35 years. TODAY. Retrieved from https://www.today.com/health/2019-birth-rates-birth-rates-us-decline-lowest-level-35-t182033.

Roberts-Douglass, K., & Curtis-Boles, H. (2013). Exploring positive masculinity development in African American men: A retrospective study. *Psychology of Men & Masculinity*, *14*(1), 7–15. https://doi.org/10.1037/a0029662

Peart, N. A., Pungello, E. P., Campbell, F. A., & Richey, T. G. (2006). Faces of fatherhood: African American young adults view the paternal role. *Families in Society: The Journal of Contemporary Social Services*, *87*(1), 71–83. https://doi.org/10.1606/1044-3894.3486

Thornton, C. (2019, November 22). *New report shows there's an African American financial literacy gap*. Black Enterprise. Retrieved from https://www.blackenterprise.com/tiaa-african-americans-financial-literacy-gap/.

TIAA Institute. (2020). *African American Personal Finance Knowledge*. Retrieved from https://www.tiaainstitute.org/about/news/african-american-personal-finance-knowledge.

Tsuchiya, K., Qian, Y., Thomas, A. Hill De Loney, E., Caldwell, C. (2018). The Effects of Multiple Dimensions of Risk and Protective Factors on Depressive Symptoms Among Nonresident African American Fathers. *American Journal of Community Psychology 62*(3–4): 464–475.

U.S. Bureau of Labor Statistics. (2019a, September 12). *Labor Force Statistics from the current population survey: Unemployment rate*.

U.S. Bureau of Labor Statistics. (2020, August). *The employment situation — August 2020*. https://www.bls.gov/news.release/pdf/empsit.pdf.

Watkins, D. C. (2012). Depression over the adult life course for African American men: Toward a framework for research and practice. *American Journal of Men's Health*, *6*(3), 194–210.

Willis, L. A. & Clark, L. F. (2007). Papa was a rolling stone and I am too: Paternal caregiving and its influence on the sexual behavior of low-income African American men. *Journal of Black Studies, 39*(4), 548–569.

Wilson, V. (2019, April 4). *Black unemployment is at least twice as high as white unemployment at the national level and in 14 states and the District of Columbia*. Economic Policy Institute. Retrieved from https://www.epi.org/publication/valerie-figures-state-unemployment-by-race/.

CHAPTER ELEVEN

For Counselors by a Counselor: Concluding Thoughts on Counseling Black Fathers

MICHAEL HANNON, PHD, LAC, NCC

The narratives included in this volume are timely, necessary, and illuminating. They offer insights for readers in at least two ways. The first is by sharing our lived experiences. It is unfortunately rare, for a variety of reasons, that Black men and fathers are encouraged and given permission to share their lives in such personal and vulnerable ways. The contributors to this book have attempted to share the breadth and depth of some of their most joyful moments and those that have made them scared, regretful, and reflective. And it is important to acknowledge that while these narratives are helpful, they are not wholly representative of Black men and fathers. Our community of Black fathers has much deeper and richer diversity in many ways that include but are not limited to educational attainment, relationship status, sexual orientation and gender identities, socioeconomic status, and ethnic identities. I remain excited and hopeful to see, read, learn, and engage with more diverse Black fathers while still celebrating the contribution this volume makes for readers.

The second type of insight this volume offers is through the contributors' clinical expertise. The Black fathers and others—who are professional counselors and counselor educators working in a variety of educational and clinical settings—provide us with their insights on suggested case conceptualization, potential treatment, and other considerations to meet the needs of Black fathers who might be at a similar juncture as they were at the time reflected in the respective chapters. The information presented is shared thoughtfully, humbly, and insightfully. In the text that follows, I provide a comprehensive set of recommendations for counseling Black fathers. It is drawn from our counseling research base, the collective clinical insight included in the previous chapters, and considerations for culturally relevant theoretical orientations, case conceptualizations, and interventions.

COUNSELING BLACK MEN AND FATHERS

The research base on effectively counseling Black fathers is inherently informed by what has been documented to be effective in counseling Black men. To say that Black men—and their mental health needs—are diverse and complex would be an understatement. What is clear is that the mental health professions have not found a consistent and effective way to encourage Black men to seek counseling support and treatment (Anderson, 2018). Hannon et al. (in press) suggested at least three factors influence men's mental health: biological factors (e.g., medical history, physical health, pre-dispositions to specific conditions), psychological factors (e.g., mental health conditions), and social factors (e.g., housing, employment). And all of these factors are influenced by how boys and men learn about masculinity and its social construction. We cannot understate that comprehensive and effective mental health care for Black fathers must consider how individual, systemic, and structural racism influence their experiences (McAdoo, 1993) and the lessons boys and men learn about what presents as authentic or real manhood and fatherhood.

Edwards (2006) indicated masculinity is a set of attributes, behaviors, and/or roles associated with being a man, arguing that men's masculinity is demonstrated in at least seven domains. They are in men's work, education, families, sexuality, health, crime, and representation. In considering masculinity for Black men in the context of their families and their fatherhood, I offer culturally relevant clinical recommendations for treating Black fathers who seek counseling support.

CULTURALLY RELEVANT CASE CONCEPTUALIZATIONS

Effective case conceptualization certainly requires counselors have a sense of their clinical or theoretical orientation(s). Brown et al. (2022) wrote that counselors' theoretical orientation provides vision, clarity, and focus that guides practice. The authors further stated, "Most helpers choose their theoretical orientation based on three considerations: the theoretical orientation of the helper's training program, the helper's life philosophy, and/or the helpers' professional experience and/or client." As a counseling professor, I have often shared with students and colleagues that counselors' theoretical orientation is a reflection of how they experience the world and the best means to facilitate therapeutic change for each client they serve.

There are hundreds of meritorious counseling theories that can guide counselors' treatment of Black father clients, and it would be both ambitious and foolish to try and present a fraction of them. Instead, I offer three important and culturally relevant counseling theories for consideration to inform how counselors can use them in case conceptualization. They are: Black Psychology, Black Existential-Humanistic Theory, and Relational Cultural Theory.

Black psychology

Scholars have noted the challenges in articulating a unified definition of Black psychology, given how diverse perspectives center Blackness as African or African-American. Cokley and Garba (2018) reminded us that Joseph White, often referred to as the father of Black psychology, described Black psychology as "... understanding the lifestyles of Black people based on their authentic experiences in this country" (p. 698). Parham et al. (1999, p. 95) cited Black/African-centered psychology as "... a dynamic manifestation of unifying African principles, values, and traditions. It is the self-conscious 'centering' of psychological analyses and applications in African realities, cultures, and epistemologies." And while there is a robust history of documented Black psychological inquiry and application than noted here, we can surmise that clinicians using Black Psychology prioritize and center clients' Black/African identity in their case conceptualizations.

Counselors drawing on Black Psychology should inherently place these fathers' Blackness at the forefront as they consider how Black fathers' presenting issue(s) may be influenced by their Black identity. Across our text, the authors wrote about a range of issues they confronted at each developmental period (e.g., pre-fatherhood; fathering their young children, adolescents; preparing them for school; helping address their mental health needs; negotiating support for neurodivergent children). Counselors should be asking themselves, *in what ways does my father clients' Blackness intersect with their presenting issues?* When considering this question and its answer(s), our prudence should lead us to consider the psychological benefits of a strong Black racial identity and the deleterious psychological and physical effects of anti-Black racism. Nobles (2013) reminded readers that people of African descent across the world have been psychologically damaged because of Eurocentric violence, colonialism, and oppression which functions a barrier to Black peoples' healthy psychological development. Black fathers are no exception. Nobles (2013, p. 236) uses derailment as a metaphor to describe anti-Black racism's influence on Black peoples' sense of self, noting:

> The complexity of psychological damage for African people can best be captured in the notion of derailment. Derailment is an important metaphor because like a train derailment, the train continues to be in motion just off its track. The cultural and psychological derailment of African people is hard to detect because African life and experience continues. The experience of human movement (or progress) continues and African people find it hard to detect that they are off their own developmental trajectory.

This is a starting point for ethically conceptualizing and responding to our Black father clients' needs and considering this significant dimension of their intersecting identities.

Black Existential-Humanistic Theory

Black and European existentialist philosophy are similar in their mutual valuing of agency and liberation for individuals. However, they differ significantly about the inequitable access for Black people to pursue their liberation because of anti-Black racism (Bassey, 2007). To this point, Vereen et al. (2017, p. 73) shared, "Liberation can be seen as the precursor and necessary foundation to accessing agency, which also has not been historically afforded to Black people." The authors also reaffirmed that European existentialist suppositions of identity, freedom, free will, and existence do not apply to the lived experiences of Black people (Vereen et al., 2017). Black Existential-Humanistic Theory can be considered a reflection and extension of Black Psychology. However, conceptualizing Black father clients' presenting issues using this theoretical orientation requires counselors to help their clients make meaning of their existence in an anti-Black world. Counselors must ask themselves and their clients, *what does it mean to be a Black man and father raising your children at this point in your life and your children's lives?*

I offer two ways to do this effectively. The first is to consider what Fanon (1967) described as *existential deviation*, or the process by which Black people simultaneously define and redefine identity, culture, and existence as a consequence of anti-Black colonialism and racism. When the Black fathers and aspiring fathers shared their narratives in the previous chapters, a Black Existentialist-Humanistic orientation would consider how frequently Black father clients have had to adjust, readjust, orient, reorient, and function in spaces and systems that do not honor, appreciate, or affirm their existence. Frequently, this comes in the form of code-switching to comport one's self and presentation in ways that are palatable or acceptable in White spaces.

The second way to draw on Black Existential-Humanistic Theory in conceptualizing Black father clients' needs is adhering to the concept of *irreducibility* in clinical practice. Perepiczka and Scholl (2012) reminded readers that Existential-Humanistic Theory, although having diverse elements, is united by the concept of *irreducibility*, or the belief that humans can only be understood as whole beings.

Hannon and Vereen (2016) urged counselors working with Black men, and by extension Black fathers, to see them as irreducible, despite how structural forces like stereotyped Black male pathology and stereotyped Black father absenteeism reduce and oversimplify Black men and their experiences. Counselors are all susceptible to racist and gendered biases which can be a predictor of unethical client care. This is particularly difficult when we acknowledge how disparate mental health care for men continues to be in the United States. However, avoiding reductionism in clinical practice can only aid in counselors' ability to provide the highest standard of care for Black father clients.

Relational-Cultural Theory (RCT)

In response to developmental theories that prioritize independence and separation, Relational-Cultural Theory posits that meaningful connections with others is at the core of human growth and development (Jordan et al., 2004). Grounded in critical feminist praxis, an overarching focus of Relational-Cultural Theory dictates that the goal of development—and thereby the requisite therapeutic work—is to become engaged in growth fostering relationships. Counselors using Relational-Cultural Theory with Black father clients will conceptualize their work, at least in part, to include assessing the extent and nature of their clients' meaningful relationships because they are predictive of therapeutic change. Clients' meaningful connections reflect relationships that are mutually empathic and empowering, and counselors' clinical work focuses on identifying those relationships that meet these criteria and being aware of and limiting relationships in which there is no mutual empathy or empowerment.

Relational-Cultural Theory has the potential to disrupt unhealthy and narrow notions of masculinity in Black father clients given its value on interconnectedness and relationships. Mahalik et al. (2003) introduced pervasive scripts that boys and men are socialized to adopt in order to be considered masculine. They included the *strong and silent* script and the *tough guy* script, both of which perpetuate that socially acceptable masculinity is demonstrated by restricted emotionality and invulnerability. Counselors' work with Black father clients would necessitate helping them identify, assess, and potentially discover new meaningful and mutually empathic and empowering relationships that illuminate the strength and growth that comes from deep connections with and interdependence on others.

CULTURALLY RELEVANT INTERVENTIONS

I conclude with recommendations for culturally relevant interventions for Black father clients, drawn from counseling research. Researchers have offered recommendations that take into account Black people's—and by extension Black fathers'—experiences with racist systems and policies that directly influence their lives. Vontress and Epp (1997) and Whaley (2001) described Black people's response to these kinds of experiences in therapy as *historical hostility* and *cultural mistrust*, both of which are patterned dispositions and responses by Black people to White sources of oppression and marginalization.

Culturally relevant and strength-based interventions that support rapport building and trust include assessment activities such as the RESPECTFUL exercise (D'Andrea & Daniels, 2001), that provides counselors an opportunity to learn and discuss with clients their most salient and often intersecting identities. Addis and Mahalik (2003) and Kiselica (2011) reminded counselors to be open to changing the context of where counseling takes place. They suggested work spaces, outdoor spaces, and other locations that allow clients to be as comfortable as possible to maximize the counseling experience.

Harper et al. (2009) offered a number of counseling interventions for Black men that include African-centered group counseling. In this case, the group is comprised of Black fathers and for Black fathers with intentional connections to Black racial identity and experiences. Washington (2018) recommended integrating hip-hop culture and rap music in individual or group counseling and Au (2005) suggested poetry therapy as a way to demonstrate interest, knowledge, and humility in learning about clients' taste in art and other forms of cultural expression. Evans et al. (2016) suggested Post-Traumatic Growth (PTG) interventions when working with Black men with race-related trauma. Vereen et al. (2013) and Solorzano and Yosso (2001) encouraged the use of culturally appropriate humor and narrative storytelling to assist in the counseling process.

While not exhaustive, these theories and interventions provide counselors with strategies and reference points to inform their work with Black father clients. It is important to note that they all place significant value on the depth and quality of the counselor–client relationship. They strike a balance between being person-centered and systems-oriented, wherein they pursue a deep and meaningful therapeutic relationship while remaining cognizant of how anti-Black racism is a pervasive force on the mental health and well-being of Black people, Black men, and Black fathers.

REFERENCES

Addis, M. E., & Mahalik, J. R. (2003). Men, masculinity, and the contexts of help seeking. *American Psychologist*, *58*(1), 5.

Anderson, M. S. (2018). Barriers to the utilization of mental Health services on college campuses by African-American students. *McNair Scholars Research Journal*, *11*(1), 1–11. Retrieved from https://commons.emich.edu/mcnair/vol11/iss1/3.

Au, W. (2005). Fresh out of school: Rap music's discursive battle with education. *The Journal of Negro Education*, *74*, 210–220.

Bassey, M. O. (2007). What Is Africana Critical Theory or Black Existential Philosophy? *Journal of Black Studies, 37*(6), 914–935. https://doi.org/10.1177/0021934705285563

Brown, N. O., Ford, Jr., D. J., Norris, J., Butler, S. K., & Filmore, J. M. (2022). Counseling theories. In S. K. Butler, A. F. Flores, & J. M. Filmore (Eds.), *21st century counseling: A multicultural and social justice approach* (pp. 92–109). San Diego: Cognella.

Cokley, K., & Garba, R. (2018). Speaking truth to power: How Black/African psychology changed the discipline of psychology. *Journal of Black Psychology*, *44*(8), 695–721. DOI: 10.177/009579841810592

D'Andrea, M., & Daniels, J. (2001). RESPECTFUL counseling: An integrative model for counselors. In D. Pope-Davis & H. Coleman (Eds.), *The intersection of race, class, and gender in multicultural counseling* (pp. 417–466). Thousand Oaks, CA: Sage.

Edwards, T. (2006). *Cultures of masculinity*. New York: Routledge.

Evans, A. M., Hemmings, C., Burkhalter, C., & Lacy, V. (2016). Responding to race related trauma: Counseling and research recommendations to promote post-traumatic growth when counseling African American males. *Journal of Counselor Preparation & Supervision*, *8*(1), 78–103.

Fanon, F. (1967). *Black skin, white masks*. New York: Grove Press.

Hannon, M. D., & Vereen, L. G. (2016). Irreducibility of Black male clients: Considerations for culturally competent counseling. *Journal of Humanistic Counseling*, *55*, 234–245. DOI: 10.1002/johc.12036.

Harper, F. D., Terry, L. M., & Twiggs, R. (2009). Counseling strategies with Black boys and Black men: Implications for policy. *Journal of Negro Education*, *78*(3), 216–232.

Jordan, J. V., Hartling, L. M., & Walker, M. (Eds.). (2004). *The complexity of connection: Writings from the Stone Center's Jean Baker Miller Training Institute*. Guilford Press.: New York.

Kiselica, M. S. (2011). Promoting positive masculinity while addressing gender role conflicts: a balanced theoretical approach to clinical work with boys and men. In C. Blazina & D. Shen-Miller (Eds.), *An international psychology of men: Theoretical advances, case studies, and clinical innovations* (pp. 127–156). New York, NY: Routledge.

Mahalik, J. R., Locke, B. D., Ludlow, L. H., Diemer, M. A., Scott, R. P., Gottfried, M., & Freitas, G. (2003). Development of the conformity to masculine norms inventory. *Psychology of Men & Masculinity*, *4*(1), 3.

McAdoo, J. L. (1993). The roles of African-American fathers: An ecological perspective. *Families in Society*, *74*(1), 28–35.

Nobles, W. (2013). Shattered consciousness, fractured identity: Black psychology and the restoration of the African psyche. *Journal of Black Psychology*, *39*(3), 232–242. DOI: 10.1177/0095798413478075

Parham, T. A., White, J. L., & Ajamu, A. (1999). *The psychology of blacks: An African-centered perspective* (3rd ed.). Englewood Cliffs, NJ: Prentice Hall.

Perepiczka, M., & Scholl, M. (2012). AHC: The heart and conscience of the counseling profession. *Journal of Humanistic Counseling*, *51*, 6–20.

Solórzano, D. G., & Yosso, T. J. (2001). Critical race and LatCrit theory and method: Counter-storytelling. *International Journal of Qualitative Studies in Education*, *14*(4), 471—495.

Vereen, L. G., Hill, N. R., & Butler, S. K. (2013). The use of humor and storytelling with African American men: Innovative therapeutic strategies for success in counseling. *International Journal for the Advancement of Counselling*, *35*(1), 57–63.

Vereen, L. G., Wines, L. A., Lemberger-Truelove, T., Hannon, M. D., Howard, N., & Burt, I. (2017). Black existentialism: Extending the discourse on meaning and existence. *Journal of Humanistic Counseling*, *56*(1), 72–84. https://doi.org/10.1002/johc.12045

Vontress, C. E., & Epp, L. (1997). Historical hostility in the African American client: implication for counseling. *Journal of Multicultural Counseling and Development*, *25*, 170–184.

Washington, A. R. (2018). Integrating hip-hop culture and rap music into social justice counseling with Black males. *Journal of Counseling and Development*, *96*, 97–105.

Whaley, A. L. (2001). Cultural mistrust and mental health services for African Americans: A review and meta-analysis. *The Counseling Psychologist*, *29*, 513–531.

Afterword: Black Fathering Counter-stories

IVORY A. TOLDSON, PHD

> Even though I don't live with my father, he still shows me what it is like to be a man by visiting every other week and keeping his word. It is important for fathers to see their children and teach them right from wrong. It is important for fathers to give their children love, and my father shows me how to do this. Young men must have positive males as role models to offer them guidance. (Toldson, 2008, p. 14).

An eighth grader named Diontre wrote these sentences in an essay he submitted to a writing contest for Black male middle and high school students called "A Mile in My Shoes." As a judge, I read Diontre's essay for content and clarity. As a researcher with a background in counseling, investigating Black male achievement, I read Diontre's essay for the qualitative context for the quantitative data that I analyzed. As a Black man and new father, I read Diontre's essay to relate my own experiences to his.

Diontre expressed how his loving relationship with his father pushed him to be a better person. However, his qualifier, "Even though I don't live with my father," gave an important context that belies conventional thinking about nonresident Black fathers. In Diontre's life, his father's consistency and honesty were more important than his residence.

Unfortunately, the spate of negative statistics about Black fathers obfuscates the simple fact that what Black fathers do is more important than who they marry or where they live. The link between father absenteeism and Black community discord surfaced over 50 years ago in the U.S. Department of Labor's Moynihan report (Ziegler, 1995). Since then, the percent of Black children being raised in single-parent homes has grown from 20 percent to 70 percent. In the United States, 31 percent of Black children have both a mother and a father in the home; 53 percent have only a mother present; 7 percent have only a father present; and 9 percent have neither parent present (Toldson, 2019).

Researchers, pundits, and culture critics have represented these figures in various ways in the media to portray a single parent crisis in the Black community. For example, in 2013 Don Lemon stated, "More than 72 percent of children in the African-American community are born out of wedlock." In the same monologue, Lemon said that the lack of role models for young Black males was "an express train right to prison."

Black Fathering and Mental Health affirms the humanity of Black fathers. The title reminds us that "father" is not just a noun. Fathering is an action that harnesses love and wisdom to inspire and empower. Dr. Hannon and his colleagues masterfully use positionality and counternarratives to illuminate the best of Black fathers. However, the book also uses keen sensibilities and astute clinical acumen to reveal the common struggles Black fathers have with responding to their children, while resisting systemic racism. Most importantly, *Black Fathering and Mental Health* offers a roadmap for being and helping Black fathers with empathy and insight.

As I reflect on my father, Dr. Ivory A. Toldson, my stepfather Dr. Imari Obadele, my daughter Makena Toldson, and my son Ivory Kaleb Toldson, I think about the possibilities of "Black Fathering and Mental Health." This is a timely volume that respects the contributions of Black scholars of the past, while capturing contemporary themes, such as intersectional identities and patriarchy. I hope mental health professionals will use this book for clinical practice, research, teaching, and policy making. I hope Black fathers, and the people who love and support them, will use this book to self-heal, self-reflect, and contribute more counter-stories that will indelibly shape the image and trajectory of Black fathering in modern society.

REFERENCES

Toldson, I. A. (2008). *Breaking barriers: Plotting the path to academic success for school-age African American males.* Congressional Black Caucus Foundation: Washington, D.C.

Toldson, I. A. (2019). *No BS (bad stats): black people need people who believe in black people enough not to believe every bad thing they hear about black people.* Leiden; Boston: Brill Sense.

Ziegler, D. (1995). Single parenting: A visual analysis. In B. J. Dickerson (Ed.), *African American single mothers: Understanding their lives and families* (pp. 80–93). Thousand Oaks, CA: Sage Publications, Inc.

Contributors

S. Kent Butler, PhD, LPC, NCC, NCSC graduated from the University of Connecticut with a PhD in educational psychology: counseling psychology. A Nationally Certified Counselor (NCC) and Nationally Certified School Counselor (NCSC), Dr. Butler serves as the 70th president of the American Counseling Association (ACA). He is ACA Fellow and currently hosts ACA's weekly vodcast "The Voice of Counseling." A National Association of Chief Diversity Officers in Higher Education Fellow (NADOHE-CDOFP), he is Full Professor of counselor education at the University of Central Florida (UCF) and former Chief Equity, Inclusion and Diversity Officer and Faculty Fellow for Inclusive Excellence.

Dr. Butler is a faculty advisor to CHI SIGMA IOTA International Honor Society (CSI), the Counselor Education Doctoral Student Organization (CEDSO), Project for Haiti Knights, and the National Association for the Advancement of Colored People (NAACP). He served as Principal Investigator for The High-Risk Delinquent and Dependent Child Educational Research Project: Situational Environmental Circumstances Mentoring Program (SEC). The grant transitioned into the UCF Young Knights Mentoring Project and supports Hungerford Elementary School students in Eatonville, FL.

Nationally, Dr. Butler is Past President for the Association for Multicultural Counseling and Development (AMCD), former ACA Governing Council Representative, and AMCD Multicultural Counseling Competencies Revisions Committee member which produced the Multicultural Social Justice Counseling Competencies (MSJCC). His research interests are Multicultural Counseling and Supervision; Social Justice; Mentoring; Black Males; and International, Group, and School Counseling.

Alfonso Ferguson, PhD, LMHC, LPC, ACS, NCC is Assistant Professor of counseling at Saybrook University, a Licensed Mental Health Counselor (LMHC) in the state of New York, a Licensed Professional Counselor (LPC) in the state of New Jersey, an Approved Clinical Supervisor (ACS), and a National Certified Counselor (NCC). Dr. Ferguson earned a doctoral degree in counseling from Montclair State University, and a master's degree in rehabilitation and mental health counseling from the University of South Florida. His counseling experience ranges from that of a counselor educator, clinical mental health counselor, and clinical consultant.

Dr. Ferguson currently owns and operates a private practice that focuses on providing culturally responsive counseling to clients from multiplymarginalized communities. He has gained a variety of experiences in individual and family counseling services to those who are experiencing psychosocial stressors, family issues, and mood disorders. He has a strong interest to work with LGBTQ+ Black Indigenous People of Color (BIPOC) living with mood disorders and psychosocial stressors. His clinical experiences include case management, inpatient and outpatient therapy, private practice owner, supervision, and consultation.

Dr. Ferguson's research has been featured in peer-reviewed journals and presented at domestic and international conferences. His research focuses on Black gay male experience, transracial adoption, and counselor education.

Gelawdiyos M. Haile, PhD, NCC is National Certified Counselor (NCC). His clinical counseling experience includes working with diverse client populations in a faith-based and private practice therapeutic setting. Dr. Haile earned a doctoral degree in counselor education and supervision from the University of Central Florida. Dr. Haile's research interests include investigating addiction recovery in diverse populations and multicultural counseling.

Amber S. Haley, PhD, LPC, LCDCI, NCC is Assistant Teaching Professor in the Department of Education and Counseling at Villanova University. She is Licensed Professional Counselor (LPC), Licensed Chemical Dependency

Counselor Intern (LCDCI), and National Certified Counselor (NCC). Her counseling experience includes work as a counselor educator, clinical mental health counselor and supervisor, and student affairs professional.

Dr. Haley is committed to the advancement of traditionally underserved and underrepresented persons from a worldview that views them as central rather than marginal to healthy human civilization. This mission is pursued via education and research focused on alleviating perceived microaggressions in cross-cultural relationships through the development of curious, humble, and culturally competent researchers and clinicians. Dr. Haley's interests also include furthering multicultural and social justice issues, counselor education and supervision competencies, and the impact of intersectionality on healthy identity development and mental wellness.

Dr. Haley earned her doctoral degree in counselor education and supervision from the University of Central Florida, a master's degree in clinical mental health counseling from Syracuse University, and a bachelor's degree in psychology with a minor in African and African Diaspora Studies from the University of Texas at Austin.

Rev. Byron L. Hannon is a semi-retired ordained elder and former senior pastor now supporting multiple multi-lingual churches and preparing up-and-coming ministers for ordination. He is also serves on the Board of Directors of Front Step, Inc., a 501c3 compassionate ministry supporting communities in North Philadelphia (PA). Prior to entering pastoral ministry, Rev. Hannon worked for over 25 years in multiple corporate settings as a Human Resources professional with the last nine years as a Director, Organization and Management Development and as a Vice President, Human Resources for an international insurance company.

Rev. Hannon's greatest passion, outside of his family, is being a discipler-mentor-coach-teacher.

Michael D. Hannon, PhD, LAC, NCC is Associate Professor of Counseling at Montclair State University, Licensed Associate Counselor (LAC), and National Certified Counselor (NCC). His counseling experience includes work as a counselor educator, clinical mental health counselor, school counselor, and student affairs professional. He is also on staff as a counselor at the Center for MARCUS in Trenton, New Jersey.

Dr. Hannon's research about Black men as fathers, otherfathers, counselor educators, and community leaders has been featured in a number of peer-reviewed journals and professional conferences. He has been a featured contributor to media outlets such as Autism Speaks, Thrive Global, Fusion, Neurodiversity Experts, and Huffington Post and awarded the 2021 Black Mental Health Educator of the Year from the Black Mental Health Symposium.

Dr. Hannon earned a doctoral degree in counselor education and supervision from The Pennsylvania State University, an educational specialist degree in school counseling services from Rider University, a master's degree in student affairs practice and a bachelor's degree in human development & family processes from the University of Delaware. Dr. Hannon and his wife, Dr. LaChan Hannon, are the co-founders of the Greater Expectations Teaching and Advocacy Center for Childhood Disabilities, Inc. (GETAC), a non-profit organization in New Jersey dedicated to supporting families raising and institutions serving children with neuro-diverse abilities and other marginalized children and families.

Tyce Nadrich, PhD, LMHC, NCC, ACS is Assistant Professor and Program Director of the Clinical Mental Health Counseling program at Molloy College. Dr. Nadrich also is Associate Dean for the School of Education and Human Services. He is Licensed Mental Health Counselor (NY), Board Certified Counselor (NCC), and Approved Clinical Supervisor (ACS). His counseling experience includes work as a counselor educator, clinical mental health counselor, and clinical supervisor for counselors in training.

Dr. Nadrich's research interests include the experiences and mental health needs of racially ambiguous people of color, Black counselors and counselor educators, and perinatal black fatherhood.

Dr. Nadrich earned a doctoral degree in counseling from Montclair State University, a master's degree in clinical mental health counseling from St. John's University, and a bachelor's degree in psychology from the City University of New York, Queens College. Dr. Nadrich currently serves as a clinician and the coordinator of clinical services at Balance Mental Health Counseling, a mental health practice that provides services to the community.

Amber R. Norman, PhD, LHMC, NCC is Clinical Faculty member at Prescott College, Licensed Mental Health Counselor (LMHC-FL), and National Certified Counselor (NCC).

Dr. Norman earned her bachelor's degree in psychology from Florida A&M University, a Historically Black College and University (HBCU) in Tallahassee, FL. She completed her graduate studies at the University of Central Florida and studied abroad at the University of South Africa in 2012. As a clinician, Amber centers her work on the health and wellness of Black, Indigenous, People of Color (BIPOC) and the queer community at large. She has worked in residential facilities, sober-living spaces and private practice supporting individuals, and groups healing from substance dependency, chronic depression, mood instability, and trauma. Her teaching and research focus on critical pedagogy, sexuality education, spirituality in counseling, and prejudice-motivated violence.

Dr. Norman is National Board of Certified Counselors Minority Fellow (2019), and she remains a fierce advocate for social justice, student mentorship, and counselor development.

Rev. Robert C. Rogers, MA, LAC, NCC has been an ordained minister in the Church of God in Christ since 1978 and currently serves as Senior Pastor at the Church of God in Christ For All Saints in Morristown, New Jersey. He is Licensed Associate Counselor (LAC) in New Jersey and National Certified Counselor (NCC). Prior to his current position, he served as a community outreach worker and organizer, financial analyst, hospital chaplain, and hospice chaplain. He has held and holds leadership positions in different ecumenical and interfaith clergy groups. He serves as a pastor and professional counselor working to organize and empower people of color to combat systemic racism and address the emotional and mental impacts of racial microaggressions and internalized oppression through counseling, psychoeducation, and spiritual liberation.

Rev. Rogers earned a master of arts in community counseling from Montclair State University, a master of business administration from Columbia University with a concentration in finance & marketing, a master of divinity in pastoral theology & human development from Princeton Theological Seminary, and a bachelor of arts in psychology & sociology from Wesleyan University in Connecticut. He is currently a doctoral candidate in counselor education at Montclair State University with a concentration in spirituality & counseling. His dissertation focuses on the stressors Black pastors experience and the impact of those stressors on pastors' mental and emotional wellness.

Sam Steen, PhD, NCC, Associate Professor, licensed Professional School Counselor, and Director of the Diversity Research Action Consortium, specializes in school counseling, group work and cultivating Black students' academic identity development. Dr. Steen was a school counselor for 10 years, and these practitioner experiences shape his research agenda, approach to teaching, and service. Currently on the faculty at George Mason University and serving as the Academic Program Coordinator, two objectives guide his scholarship: (1) to further develop creative and culturally sustaining school-based counseling interventions that improve student achievement; including The Achieving Success Everyday Group Model (ASE Group Model) designed to promote social emotional and academic development for students of color and (2) to explore issues related to the training and preparation of pre-service counselors and school counselors in the local, regional, and national community.

Dr. Steen is Fellow for the Association for Specialists in Group Work, a division of the American Counseling Association. Dr. Steen is also the recipient of the Al Dye Research Award and the Professional Advancement Award both from ASGW recognizing his outstanding efforts advancing the field of group work though research and development of a new and innovative strategies for schools, families, and underrepresented communities. Recently, Dr. Steen is serving as a principal investigator on a major project that is awarded by the National Science Foundation which aims to advance programs, knowledge, and skills targeting Black male middle school students for better accessibility, and higher likelihood for success, in Algebra 1 and future STEM-related careers.

Ivory Toldson, PhD is National Director of education innovation and research for the NAACP, Professor of counseling psychology at Howard University and Editor-in-Chief of The Journal of Negro Education. Previously, Dr. Toldson was appointed by President Barack Obama to devise national strategies to sustain and expand federal support to HBCUs as the executive director of the White House Initiative on Historically Black Colleges and Universities (WHIHBCUs). He also served as president and CEO of the QEM Network and contributing education editor for The Root, where he debunked some of the most pervasive myths about African-Americans in his "Show Me the Numbers" column.

Dr. Toldson is the Executive Editor of the Journal of Policy Analysis and Research, published by the Congressional Black Caucus Foundation, Inc. He is also the author of Brill Bestseller, No BS (Bad Stats): Black People Need People Who Believe in Black People Enough Not to Believe Every Bad Thing They Hear about Black People. Dr. Toldson is ranked among the nation's top education professors as a member of Education Week's Edu-Scholar Public Influence Rankings; an annual list recognizes university-based scholars across the nation who are champions in shaping educational practice and policy.

Linwood G. Vereen, PhD, NCC, LPC is Associate Professor in the Department of Counseling and College Student Personnel at Shippensburg University of Pennsylvania. Dr. Vereen serves as the current editor of the Journal of Humanistic Counseling and has scholarly interests in leadership, Black existentialism, group work, humanistic counseling, and student athlete development. He is a past recipient of the Locke-Paisley Mentoring award from the Association of Counselor Education and Supervision (ACES) and is a longstanding member of the American Counseling Association (ACA). As a leader in the counseling profession he has served as the president of the Idaho Counseling Association, president of the Association for Humanistic Counseling and been the western Regional Chair for the American Counseling Association.

In addition to his role as an educator, Dr. Vereen has served as a professional counselor, advocate, consultant, and child custody evaluator. He works with a diverse group of persons and students as an instructor, advisor, mentor, and consultant.

Dr. Vereen is the first Black man to earn his PhD in counselor education from the University of Nevada Reno. He is a native of Connecticut where he earned his bachelor's degree while being a scholarship member of the football team. He went on to also earn a master's degree in counseling psychology from the University of Connecticut.

Rodney N. West, MA is School Counselor at Piscataway High School (PHS) in New Jersey. At PHS, Mr. West is also an advisor for 50 Strong, a Title I program focused on building social and emotional wellness in young men of color. He also assists in the School Counseling program at Montclair State University as a Cooperating Counselor.

Mr. West earned his bachelor's degree in business administration with a concentration in finance from the University of Delaware. Rodney worked in the finance industry for 15 years as Business Analyst and Project Manager before deciding to change careers and earning his master's degree in school counseling from Capella University.

Eric Williams, PhD, LCMHCS (NC), LMFT (NC), LPC (GA), NCC is Assistant Professor of Clinical Mental Health Counseling at Huntington University, Licensed Clinical Mental Health Counselor Supervisor (LCMHCS), Licensed Professional Counselor (LPC), Licensed Marriage & Family Therapist (LMFT), and Nationally Certified Counselor (NCC). He is also a Christian, husband of 15 years, father of twin boys on the autism spectrum, a "girl dad" to his daughter, and a US Army veteran.

Dr. Williams' current counseling experiences include military installations, clinical supervisor, private practice, and as a counselor educator. He is the owner of Coastal Family Services, PLLC in Fayetteville, NC and serves on the board of directors for both Autism Society of Cumberland County in Fayetteville, NC and Mariposa School for Children with Autism in Cary, NC.

He has several blogs featured on popular websites like Yahoo Finance, Yahoo Parenting, YourTango, PopSugar, and Autism Society of North Carolina. Additionally, he has spoken at several conferences on the topics of autism and parenting.

Dr. Williams earned his doctoral degree in counselor education and supervision from Regent University and his master's degree in marriage and family therapy from Valdosta State University. He is a Georgia native and true Bulldawgs fan!

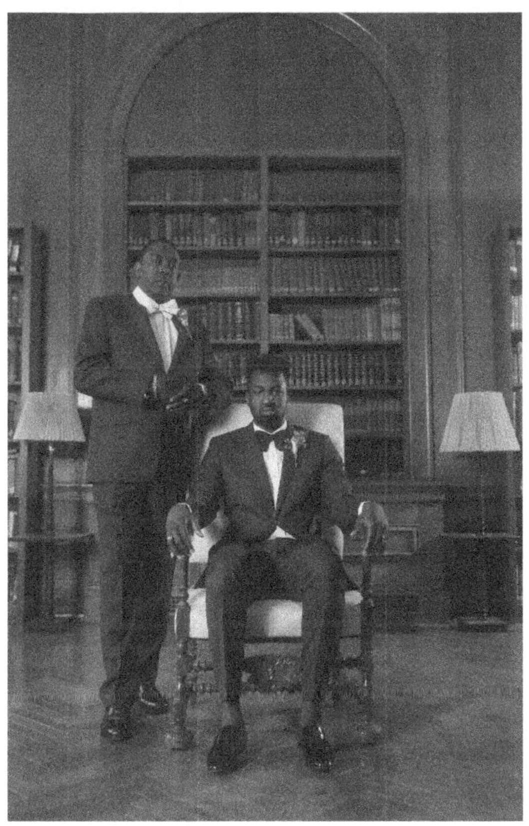

Picture 1. Alfonso Ferguson, Sr. and Alfonso Ferguson, Jr.

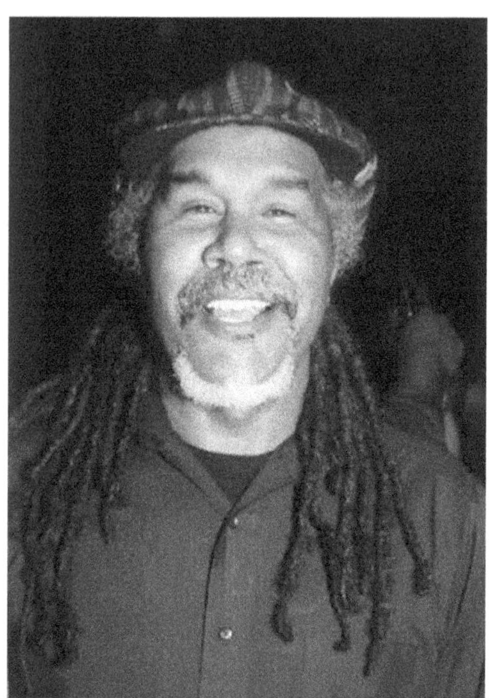

Picture 2. Coach Horace Ruddock

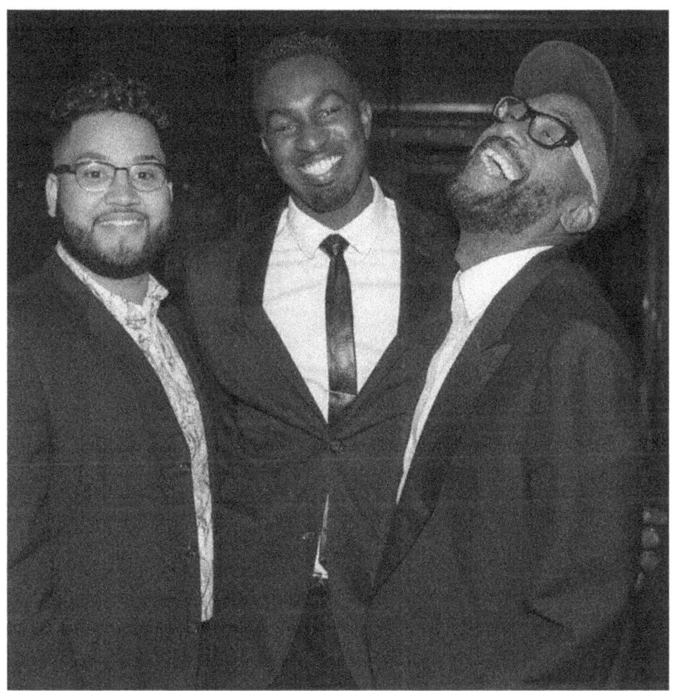

Picture 3. Daton Haywood Ferguson, Alfonso Ferguson, Jr., and Gregory Russell aka Nana

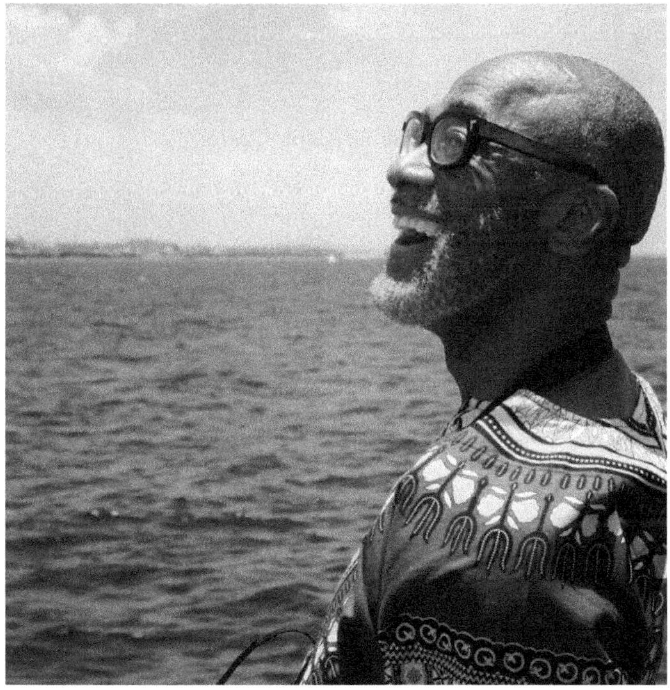

Picture 4. Gregory Russell aka Nana

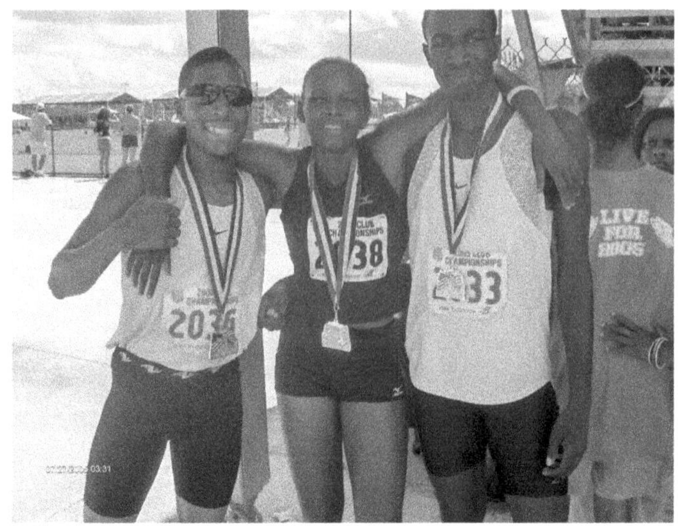

Picture 5. John Bullock, Deandra Ford, and Alfonso Ferguson, Jr.

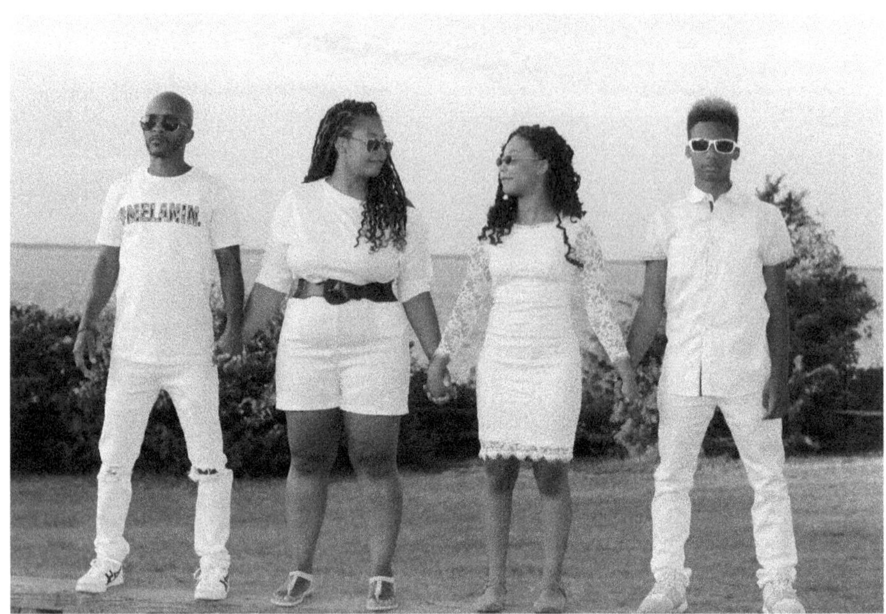

Picture 6. Michael, LaChan, Nile, and Avery Hannon

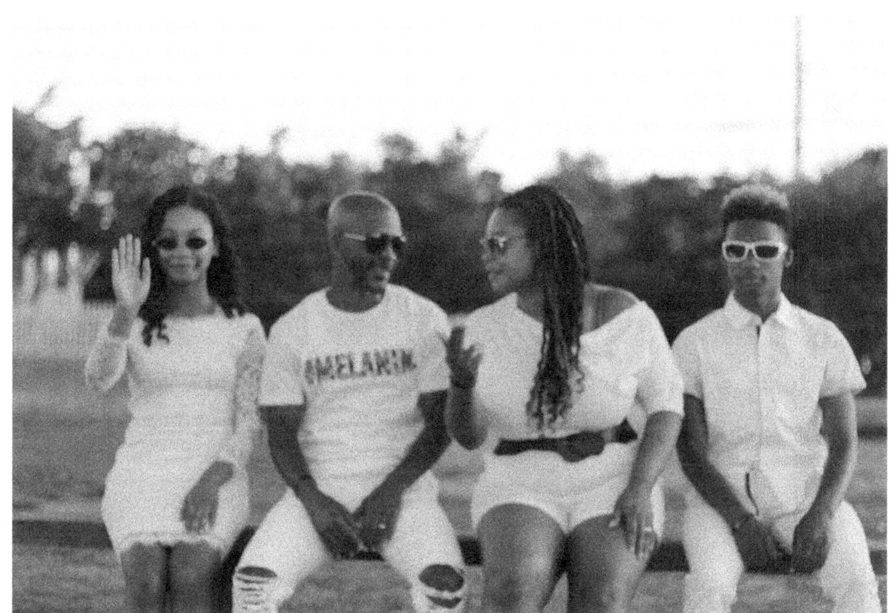

Picture 7. Nile, Michael, LaChan, and Avery Hannon

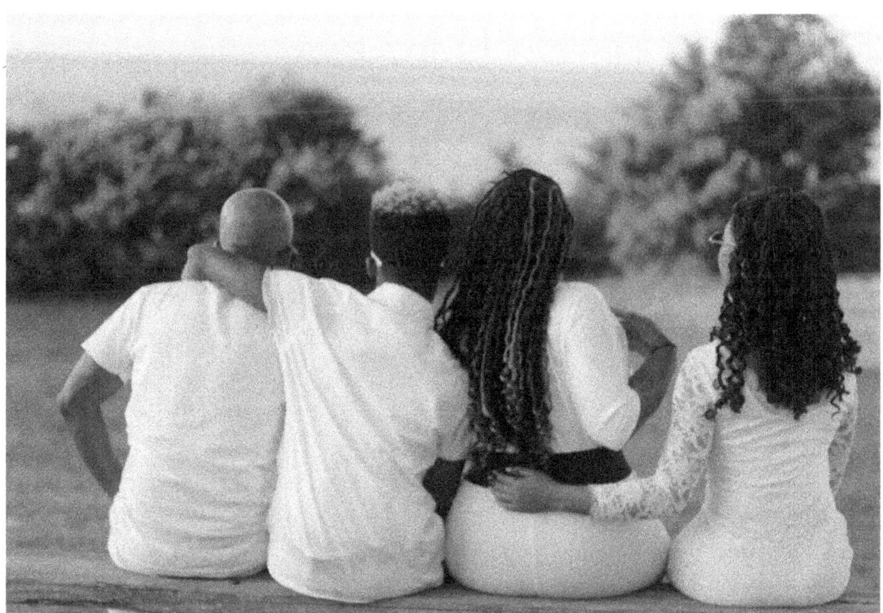

Picture 8. Michael, Avery, LaChan, and Nile Hannon

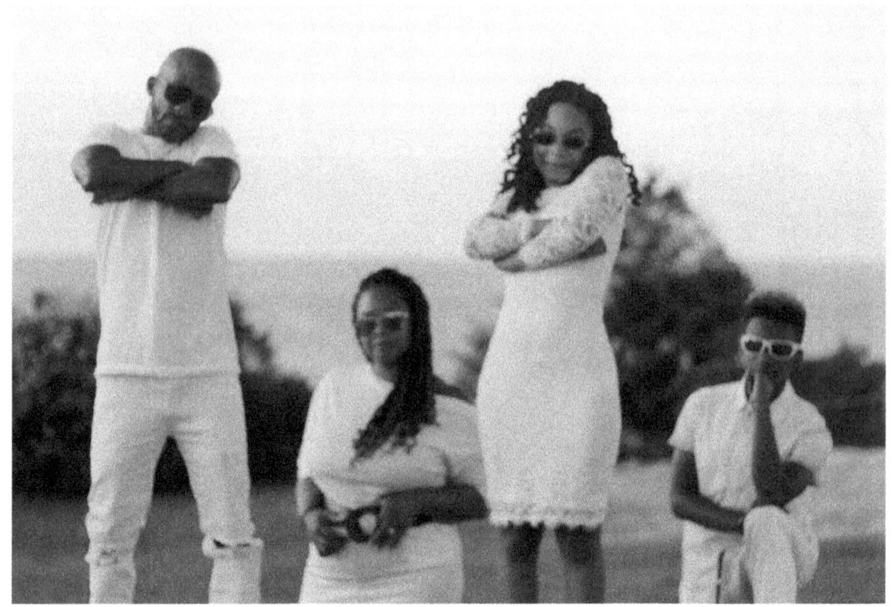

Picture 9. Michael, LaChan, Nile, and Avery Hannon

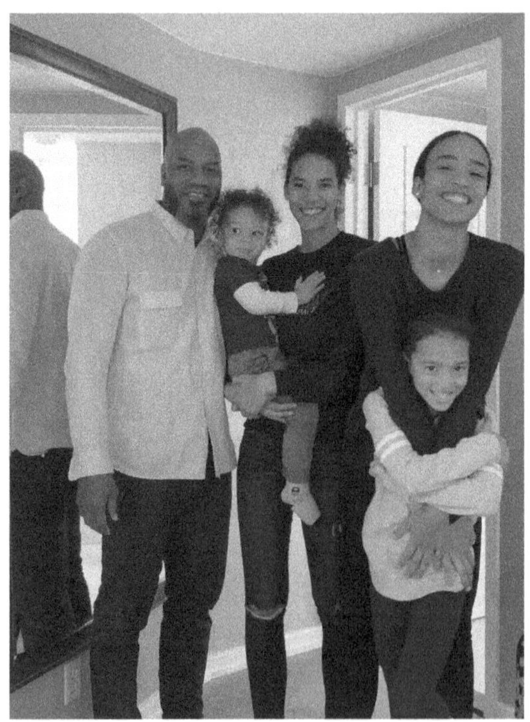

Picture 10. Linwood Vereen, Maxwell Hill-Vereen, Kenady Vereen, Ryan Vereen, and Maelee Hill-Vereen

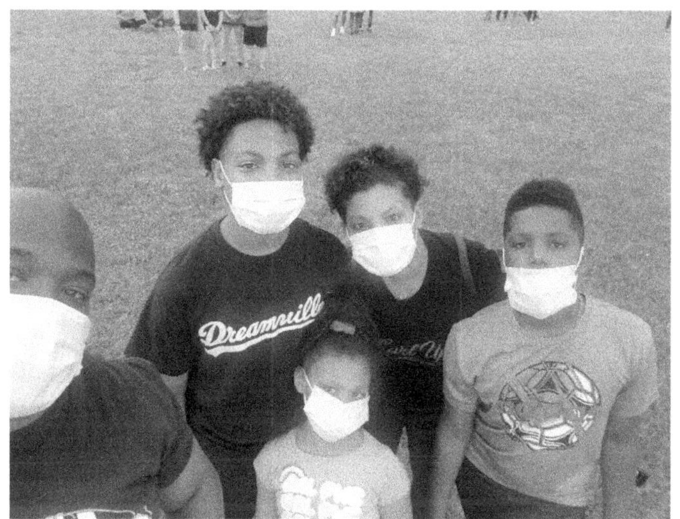

Picture 11. Rodney, Xavier, Sydney, Nicole, and Tyler West

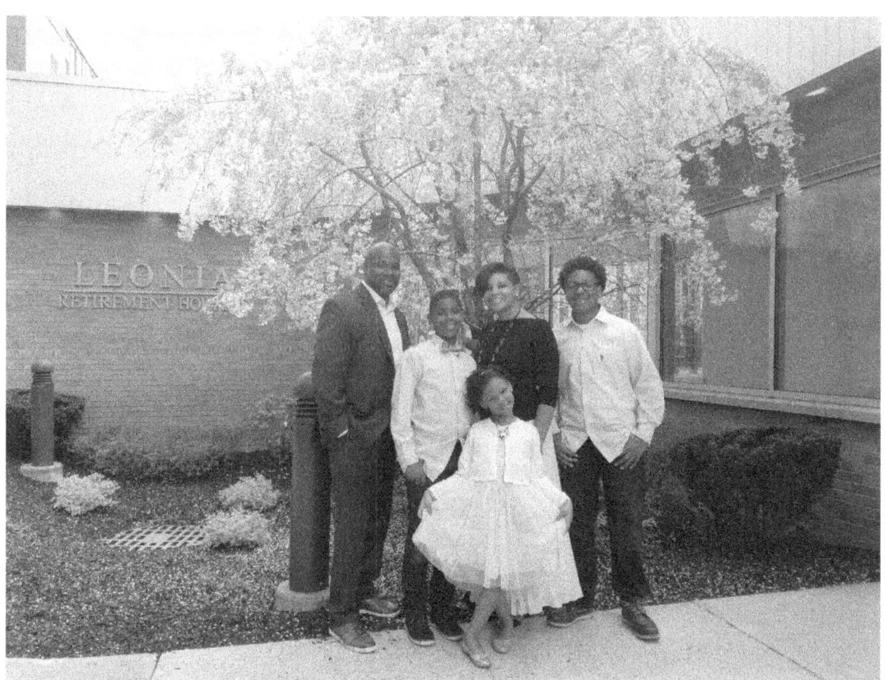

Picture 12. Rodney, Tyler, Sydney, Nicole, and Xavier West

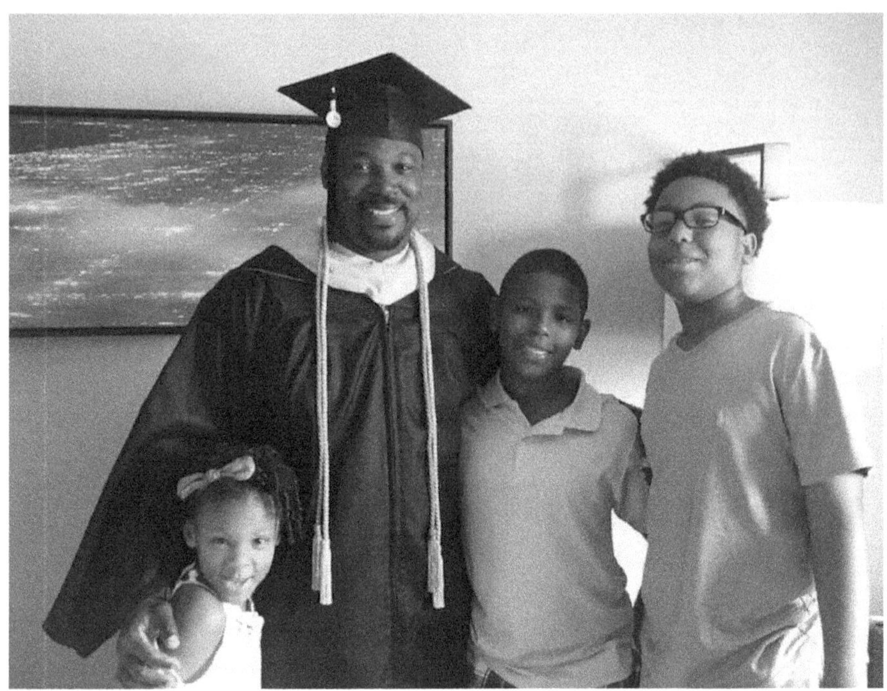

Picture 13. Sydney, Rodney, Tyler, and Xavier West

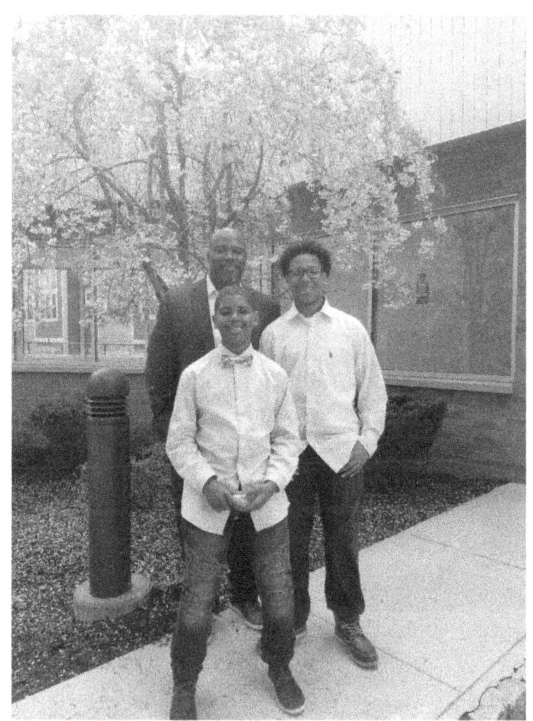

Picture 14. Rodney, Tyler, and Xavier West

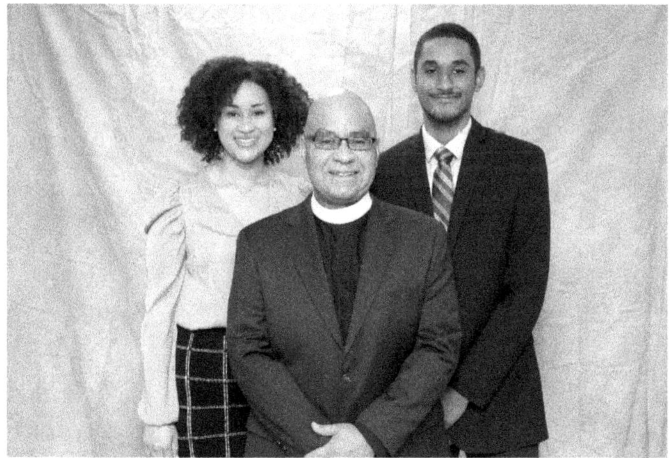

Picture 15. Khiana, Robert, and Kendall Rogers

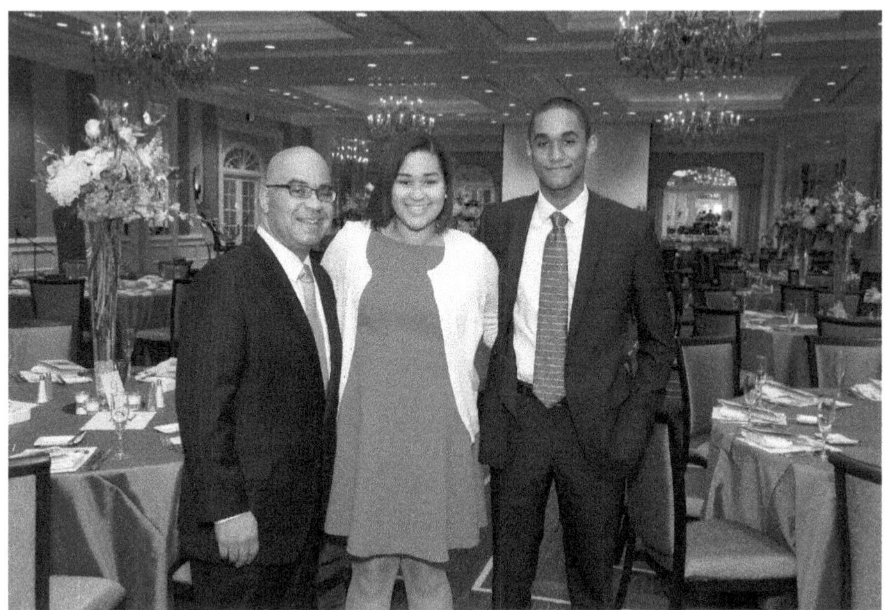

Picture 16. Robert, Khiana, and Kendall Rogers (December 2014)

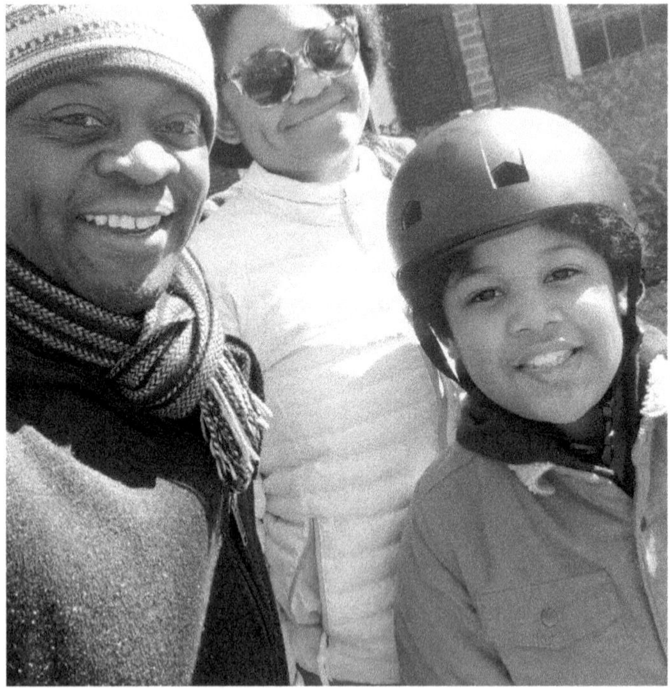

Picture 17. Sam, Madeleine Claire Santella, and Tristan Oliver Santella Steen

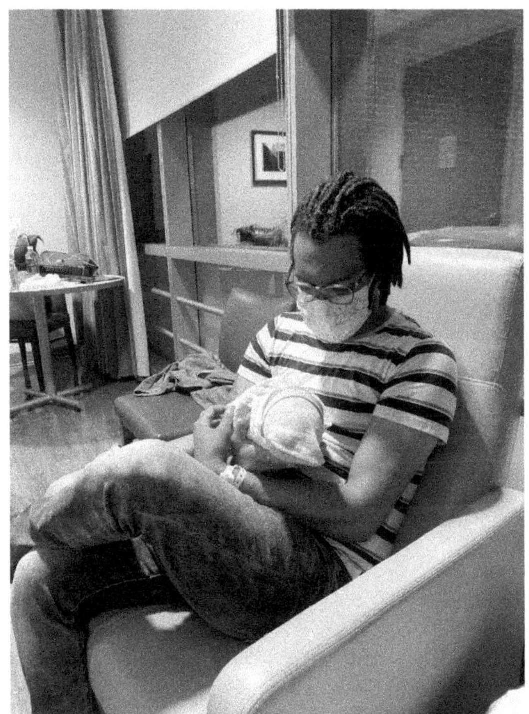

Picture 18. Tyce and Lily Nadrich

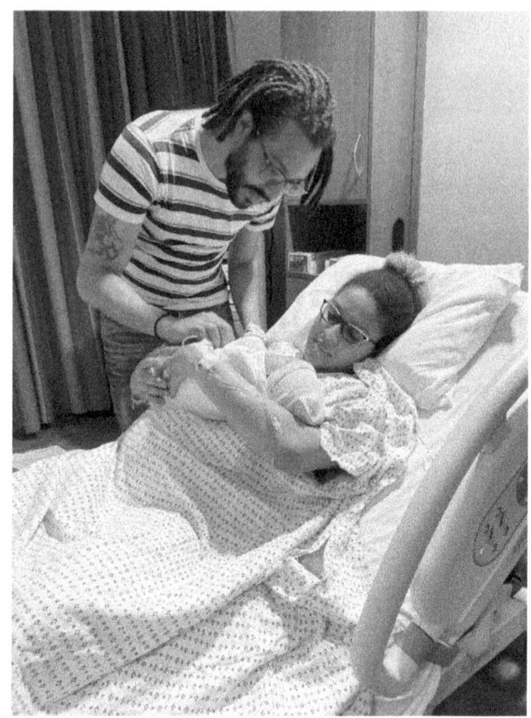

Picture 19. Tyce, Josie, and Lily Nadrich

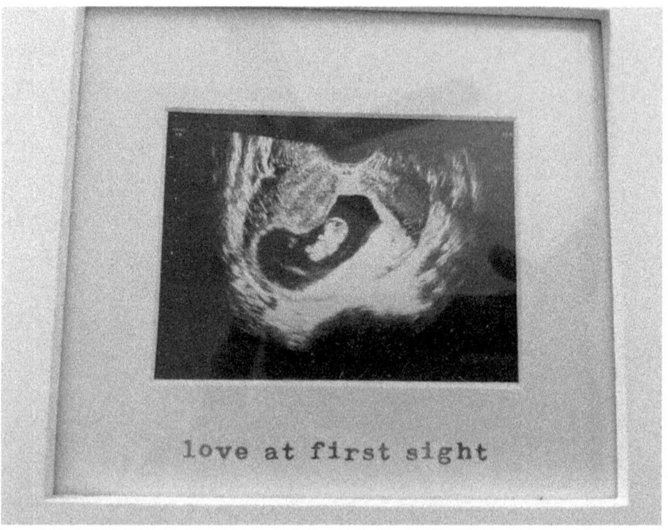

Picture 20. Lily Nadrich Ultrasound

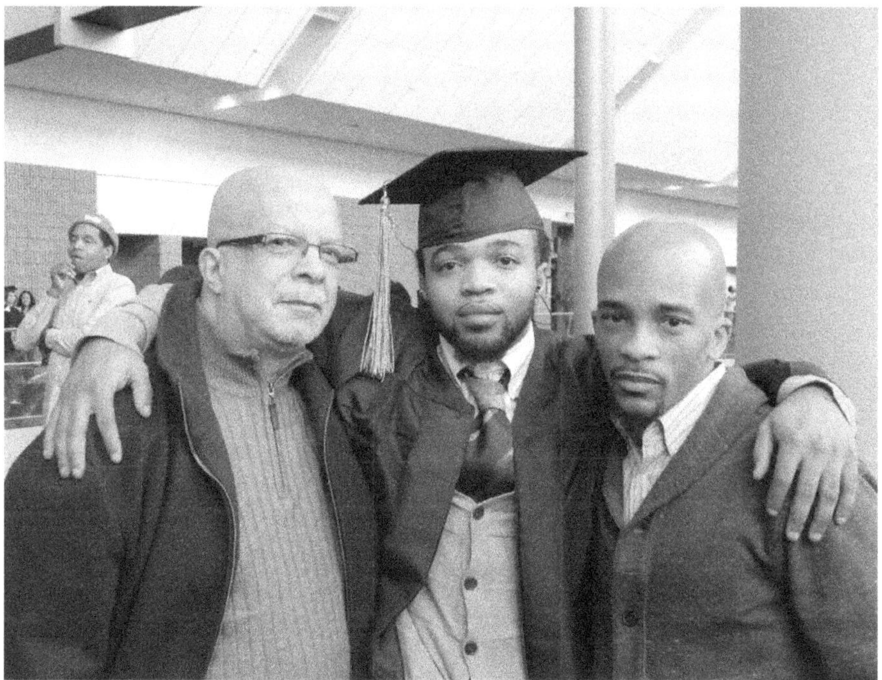
Picture 21. Byron, Nathan, and Michael Hannon

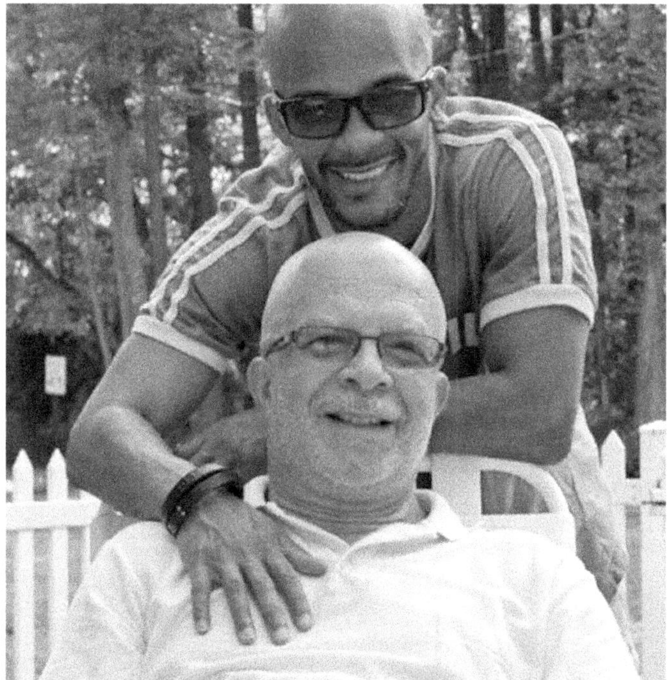
Picture 22. Michael and Byron Hannon

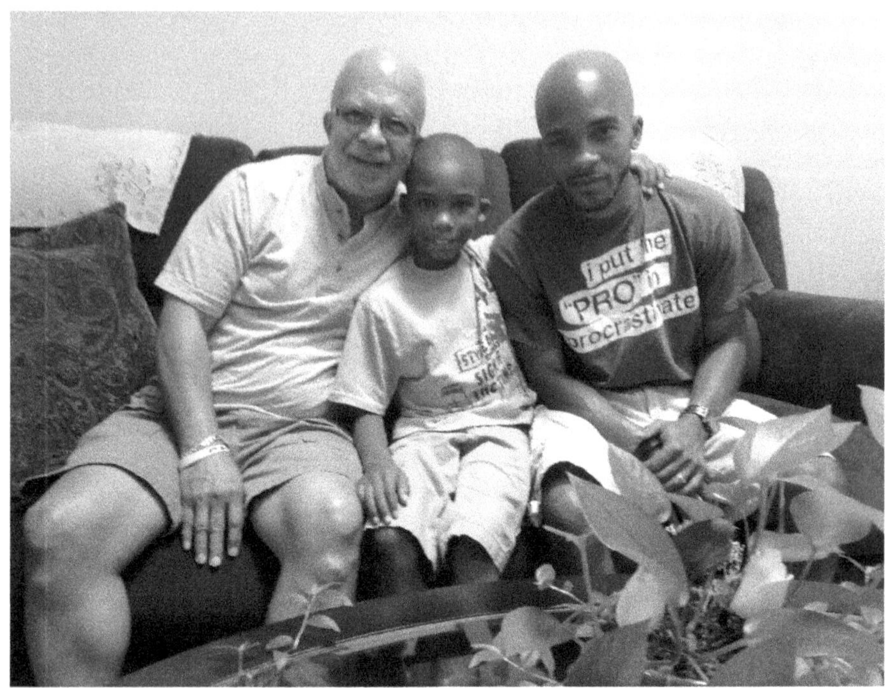

Picture 23. Byron, Avery, and Michael Hannon

www.ingramcontent.com/pod-product-compliance
Ingram Content Group UK Ltd.
Pitfield, Milton Keynes, MK11 3LW, UK
UKHW020615180726
13836UKWH00010B/2492

9 781433 193095